IMMUNOLOGIC ADJUVANT RESEARCH

IMMUNOLOGIC ADJUVANT RESEARCH

ANTONIO H. BENVENUTO
EDITOR

Nova Biomedical Books
New York

Copyright © 2009 by Nova Science Publishers, Inc.

All rights reserved. No part of this book may be reproduced, stored in a retrieval system or transmitted in any form or by any means: electronic, electrostatic, magnetic, tape, mechanical photocopying, recording or otherwise without the written permission of the Publisher.

For permission to use material from this book please contact us:
Telephone 631-231-7269; Fax 631-231-8175
Web Site: http://www.novapublishers.com

NOTICE TO THE READER

The Publisher has taken reasonable care in the preparation of this book, but makes no expressed or implied warranty of any kind and assumes no responsibility for any errors or omissions. No liability is assumed for incidental or consequential damages in connection with or arising out of information contained in this book. The Publisher shall not be liable for any special, consequential, or exemplary damages resulting, in whole or in part, from the readers' use of, or reliance upon, this material. Any parts of this book based on government reports are so indicated and copyright is claimed for those parts to the extent applicable to compilations of such works.

Independent verification should be sought for any data, advice or recommendations contained in this book. In addition, no responsibility is assumed by the publisher for any injury and/or damage to persons or property arising from any methods, products, instructions, ideas or otherwise contained in this publication.

This publication is designed to provide accurate and authoritative information with regard to the subject matter covered herein. It is sold with the clear understanding that the Publisher is not engaged in rendering legal or any other professional services. If legal or any other expert assistance is required, the services of a competent person should be sought. FROM A DECLARATION OF PARTICIPANTS JOINTLY ADOPTED BY A COMMITTEE OF THE AMERICAN BAR ASSOCIATION AND A COMMITTEE OF PUBLISHERS.

Library of Congress Cataloging-in-Publication Data

Immunologic adjuvant research / editor, Antonio Benvenuto.
     p. ; cm.
  Includes bibliographical references and index.
  ISBN 978-1-60692-399-3 (softcover)
  1. Immunological adjuvants. I. Benvenuto, Antonio, 1945-
  [DNLM: 1. Adjuvants, Immunologic--pharmacokinetics. 2. Immunotherapy, Active--methods. QW 800 I324 2009]
     QR187.3.I46   2009
     571.9'645--dc22
                                                                         2008050550

Published by Nova Science Publishers, Inc. ✢ *New York*

Contents

Preface vii

Chapter 1 Adjuvants in Cancer Vaccination 1
Ralf Kircheis and Andreas Nechansky

Chapter 2 TLR Agonists as Immune Adjuvants 47
Yanal Murad and Bara Sarraj

Chapter 3 Modulating Immune Response with CpG-Oligodeoxynucleotide through the Skin 71
Joe Inoue and Yukihiko Aramaki

Chapter 4 Immunopotentiating Reconstituted Influenza Virosomes as Safe and Potent Antigen-Delivery System for Synthetic Peptides in Vaccine Development 87
Claudia A. Daubenberger, Gerd Pluschke, Rinaldo Zurbriggen, and Nicole Westerfeld

Expert Commentary

Vaccine Adjuvants: Priorities and Challenges 97
Ali M. Harandi and Ole F. Olesen

Short Communication

The Involvement of Interleukin-6 in the Augmentation of Immune Response by Immunologic Adjuvants 105
Masahiko Mihara and Hiroto Yoshida

Index 113

Preface

In immunology, an adjuvant refers to any agent that stimulates the immune system and thus, increases the response to a vaccine. Optimal conditions for effective processing of the antigen are provided by the appropriate adjuvants. This book discusses the role of such immunologic adjuvants in diseases such as cancer, their clinical use and their potential future applications. Cancer is often associated with an increasingly impaired immune response against a tumor. Escape mechanisms of the tumor affect the ability of the immune system to build up an effective response against the growing tumor. The roles of such adjuvants in cancer vaccinations are described. Toll like receptors (TLRs) are part of the innate immune system. They are considered as major targets for the development of agonists that could serve as adjuvants and agents of immunotherapy. The development of TLR agonists for clinical use are discussed as well. CpG-ODN (oligodeoxynucleotide) is described as well as how it could be effective as an adjuvant for humoral and cellular immunities. Additionally, a transcutaneous vaccination as an effective approach for the development of tumor vaccines is explained. The development of effective vaccines for malaria, tuberculosis and HIV represents one of the most important scientific public health challenges of our time. Novel concepts in malaria proteins are examined as well as recent advances in the design of synthetic vaccine candidates and antigen delivery systems based on immuno-potentiating reconstituted influenza virosomes. The majority of vaccines presently under investigation represents highly pure recombinant proteins or subunits of pathogens and hence lacks most of the features of the original pathogens. Thus, the development of safe and potent immunologic adjuvants that can enhance and direct vaccine-specific immunity is urgently needed. Aluminum hydroxide (alum) is currently the only vaccine adjuvant approved for human use worldwide. Thus, recent developments in immunology are examined as well as Toll-like receptors and other innate immune receptors. Finally, interleukin-6 plays a crucial role in CFA-augmented immune reactions. Thus, studies that shed light on the involvement of interleukin-6 in the augmentation of immune response by immunologic adjuvants are explained.

Chapter 1 - Cancer is often associated with an increasingly impaired immune response against the tumor. Escape mechanisms of the tumor - such as loss of antigen expression, reduced major histocombatibility complex (MHC) expression, absence of co-stimulatory molecules, suppression of anti-tumor immune responses by regulatory cells, and alterations in the cytokine profile - affect the ability of the immune system to build up an effective response against the growing tumor. Consequently, the tumor has often induced immunological tolerance which needs to be broken by immune therapy. Tumor associated antigens are recognized by T-cells or antibodies which subsequently mediate tumor cell destruction indicating that the use of the appropriate target antigen(s) - combined with a balanced cytokine profile – have the potential to convert cancer vaccines into effective anti-cancer therapeutics. In order to increase the immunogenicity of antigens, a variety of adjuvants are currently studied for cancer vaccination. The term adjuvant is used for any agent with the potential to increase the humoral or cellular immune response to an antigen. Appropriate adjuvants are supposed to provide the necessary milieu and the optimal conditions for effective processing and presentation of the antigen by the antigen presenting cells (APCs) to the T cells. In this context the antigen formulation and the cytokine balance have been identified as pivotal factors for effective activation. To optimize the magnitude and quality of the specific immune response, suitable vaccine adjuvants are required, and much effort is spent identifying new, effective and non-toxic adjuvant formulations. The major attribute of a successful adjuvant is the induction of a long-term, potent and safe immune response. The choice of any adjuvant reflects a compromise between a requirement for immunogenicity and an acceptable low level of adverse reactions.

This article reviews the state-of-the-art in the adjuvant field, and explores future directions of adjuvant development with respect to the different approaches in cancer therapy, ranging from cytokine gene-modified tumor cells to synthetic vaccine formulations.

Chapter 2 - The immune system can be broadly divided into innate and adaptive, bridged by antigen-presenting cells, like dendritic cells. While the adaptive immunity is specific and requires antigen presentation, the innate immune system recognizes foreign pathogens in a non-specific manner, and then responds through effectors like cytokines. Toll like receptors (TLRs) are part of the innate immune system, and they belong to the pattern recognition receptors (PRR) family, which is designed to recognize and bind certain molecules that are restricted to pathogens, like LPS and CpG. Different TLR signals converge through few common adapter proteins to relay their signals, a process that results in the activation of several genes essential for mounting an immune response. The wide distribution of TLRs on hematopoietic and non-hematopoietic cells, and their high potential for activating the host immune system makes TLR ligands great adjuvant candidates. They will elicit their function on a wide variety of cells, and stimulate both the innate and adaptive immune systems. Thus, TLRs are considered as major targets for the development of agonists that could serve as adjuvants and agents of immunotherapy. Several of these TLR agonists, including TLR2, TLR4, TLR7 and TLR9 agonists are being developed and tested in clinical trials. This chapter reviews the development of these agonists for clinical use, and potential future applications.

Chapter 3 - Unmethylated CpG dinucleotides flanked by certain bases (CpG-motif), which are present in bacterial DNA, have been shown to be immunostimulatory. Previous studies have found that both bacterial CpG-motifs and synthetic oligodeoxynucleotides containing a CpG-motif (CpG-ODN) activate cells such as B-cells, macrophages and dendritic cells (DC), through toll-like receptor-9 (TLR-9). Signaling through TLR-9 has been shown to lead to the secretion of large amounts of cytokines such as type-I IFN and IL-12.

These cytokines act on T cells inducing the production of cytokines, primarily IFN-γ. CpG-ODN also induces the production of great numbers of CTLs which have anti-tumor effects. Consequently, CpG-ODN could be effective as an adjuvant for humoral and cellular immunities.

The authors have demonstrated that the administration of CpG-ODN through the skin induced a Th1-type immune response and this suggests that the skin is a potential site for vaccination. Additionally, the transcutaneous vaccination of a tumor-antigen and CpG-ODN in combination with a COX-2 inhibitor was effective in inducing antigen-specific anti-tumor immunity *in vivo*. These results suggest that this transcutaneous vaccination is an effective approach for the development of tumor vaccines.

The authors have also reported that administration of CpG-ODN through the skin may shift the immune response from type Th2 to Th1 and drastically attenuate the production of IgE in mice undergoing an IgE-type immune response. The application of CpG-ODN remarkably changed the immune response from type Th2 to Th1 in NC/Nga mice which spontaneously developed atopic dermatitis (AD)-like symptoms and high-Th2-immune responses. These results suggest CpG-ODN is effective for immunotherapy in patients with AD, which is characterized by Th2-dominated inflammation.

In summary, vaccination with CpG-ODN through the skin is a very simple and cost effective strategy for the development of tumor vaccine and immunotherapy in patients with AD and may be readily achievable.

Chapter 4 - The development of effective vaccines for malaria, tuberculosis and HIV represents one of the most important scientific public health challenges of our time. One possible approach is based on subunit vaccines that utilize well defined antigens for which there is evidence of protective immunity from epidemiological data in the field or animal challenge models. In malaria vaccine development, it is generally accepted that an effective subunit vaccine will target antigens of several developmental stages of the parasite *Plasmodium falciparum*. Currently, the development of subunit vaccines is hampered by their poor immunogenicity and lack of suitable antigen delivery systems driving appropriate immune responses in humans. Most importantly, the recombinant proteins or synthetic peptides delivered have to mimic closely the corresponding native malaria protein to induce effective antibody responses. Here we focus on novel concepts in malaria vaccine development highlighting recent advances in the design of synthetic vaccine candidates and antigen delivery systems based on immuno-potentiating reconstituted influenza virosomes.

Expert Commentary - The majority of vaccines presently under investigation represents highly pure recombinant proteins or subunits of pathogens and hence lacks most of the features of the original pathogens such as the inherent immunostimulatory property. Thus, the development of safe and potent immunologic adjuvants that can enhance and direct vaccine-specific immunity is urgently needed.

With few exceptions, aluminum hydroxide (alum) is currently the only vaccine adjuvant approved for human use worldwide. Although alum is effective at generating strong antibody response following repeated administration, it fails to elicit T cell immunity, which is essential to combat several life-threatening infections and cancers. This calls for rational design of prospective vaccine adjuvants that can establish protective immunity with fewer vaccinations with less injected material, through long-lasting antibody and cell-mediate immune responses. Recent developments in immunology, including the discovery of Toll-like receptors and other innate immune receptors with the capacity of bridging innate and adaptive immunity as well as novel delivery systems have offered new opportunities to delve into this avenue.

Despite the fact that the efficacy of new or improved vaccines depends critically on the accompanying adjuvants, research on vaccine adjuvants has so far received little attention as an independent scientific priority from most of the major research funding agencies and policy makers. At the same time, adjuvant research and development is currently spread over a wide number of highly diverse organizations, including large commercial companies, small biotech enterprises as well as publicly-funded research organizations and academia.

More efforts are therefore needed to highlight the importance of adjuvants on the global research agenda, but also to encourage collaboration and flow of information between different stakeholders. The European Commission has recognized the necessity to foster collaborative research, and has supported the development of novel or improved vaccines through successive Framework Programmes. Concurrent development and testing of new adjuvants has been an integrated part of these activities, and this has created a significant momentum in adjuvant research and development. Future challenges will be to keep up the momentum, to share available knowledge about adjuvants across sectors, and to facilitate access to the most promising adjuvants.

Short Communication - In this article, we summarized studies that shed light on the involvement of IL-6 in immune reactions augmented by immunologic adjuvants such as complete Freund's adjuvant (CFA) and aluminum hydroxide (alum). Firstly, we considered humoral antibody responses. In one study, immunization with DNP-KLH plus CFA induced high blood IL-6 levels and augmented anti-DNP antibody production compared with DNP-KLH alone. Blockade of IL-6 signaling by anti-IL-6 receptor (IL-6R) antibody dose-dependently suppressed the increase in CFA-augmented anti-DNP antibody production. In another study, immunization with OVA plus alum augmented anti-OVA IgE production, but IL-6 production was not detectable and anti-IL-6R antibody did not suppress IgE production. Secondly, we considered cellular immune responses. Delayed-type hypersensitivity (DTH), an antigen-specific, cell-mediated immune reaction, was elicited by CFA plus antigen. Spleen cells from immunized mice produced IL-2 and IFN-γ when stimulated by antigen (mycobacteria), suggesting that CFA induces Th1 differentiation. Anti-IL-6R antibody significantly suppressed the DTH reaction and the production of IL-2 and IFN-γ by spleen cells, suggesting that IL-6 is needed for the DTH reaction and for Th1 differentiation. Th17, a recently discovered helper T cell that produces IL-17, is attracting attention for its role in autoimmune disease models. To study this, collagen-induced arthritis (CIA) was induced by two immunizations with type II collagen plus CFA. Th1 cells and Th17 cells were induced in spleen in this model. When injected at the first immunization, anti-IL-6R antibody suppressed the onset of arthritis and the induction of Th1 and Th17 cells. In conclusion, IL-6 plays a crucial role in CFA-augmented immune reactions, but not in alum-augmented ones. Since CFA and alum evoke different immune responses, and this should be taken into account when using them as adjuvants.

In: Immunologic Adjuvant Research
Editor: Antonio H. Benvenuto

ISBN 978-1-60692-399-3
© 2009 Nova Science Publishers, Inc.

Chapter 1

Adjuvants in Cancer Vaccination

Ralf Kircheis[1] and Andreas Nechansky[2]

(1) Meridian Biopharmaceuticals GmbH, Brunner Strasse 69, A-1230 Vienna, Austria
(2) Vela Laboratories, Brunner Strasse 69 / Obj. 3, A-1230 Vienna, Austria

Abstract

Cancer is often associated with an increasingly impaired immune response against the tumor. Escape mechanisms of the tumor - such as loss of antigen expression, reduced major histocombatibility complex (MHC) expression, absence of co-stimulatory molecules, suppression of anti-tumor immune responses by regulatory cells, and alterations in the cytokine profile - affect the ability of the immune system to build up an effective response against the growing tumor. Consequently, the tumor has often induced immunological tolerance which needs to be broken by immune therapy. Tumor associated antigens are recognized by T-cells or antibodies which subsequently mediate tumor cell destruction indicating that the use of the appropriate target antigen(s) - combined with a balanced cytokine profile – have the potential to convert cancer vaccines into effective anti-cancer therapeutics. In order to increase the immunogenicity of antigens, a variety of adjuvants are currently studied for cancer vaccination. The term adjuvant is used for any agent with the potential to increase the humoral or cellular immune response to an antigen. Appropriate adjuvants are supposed to provide the necessary milieu and the optimal conditions for effective processing and presentation of the antigen by the antigen presenting cells (APCs) to the T cells. In this context the antigen formulation and the cytokine balance have been identified as pivotal factors for effective activation. To optimize the magnitude and quality of the specific immune response, suitable vaccine adjuvants are required, and much effort is spent identifying new, effective and non-toxic adjuvant formulations. The major attribute of a successful adjuvant is the induction of a long-term, potent and safe immune response. The choice of

---

[1] Tel.: +43-699-13143113 FAX: +43-1-890 597910 , e-mail: r.kircheis@meridian-biopharm.at web site: www.meridian-biopharm.at.

any adjuvant reflects a compromise between a requirement for immunogenicity and an acceptable low level of adverse reactions.

This article reviews the state-of-the-art in the adjuvant field, and explores future directions of adjuvant development with respect to the different approaches in cancer therapy, ranging from cytokine gene-modified tumor cells to synthetic vaccine formulations.

Keywords: *adjuvant, alum, AS02, BCG, carbohydrate-specific immune response, CpG, cytokines, Detox-B, ENHANZYN, GM-CSF, heat shock protein, IC31, IL-2, IL-12, IFNα, ISCOMS, LPS, MPL, MF59, SialylTn, QS-21*

Introduction

An adjuvant is defined as a product that increases or modulates the immune response against an antigen (Ag). According to this general definition the ideal adjuvant increases the potency of the immune response while being non-toxic and safe. Although dozens of different adjuvants have been shown to be effective in preclinical and clinical studies, only aluminum-based salts (Alum) and squalene-oil-water emulsion (MF59) have been approved for human use until now. Moreover, for the development of therapeutic vaccines for treatment of cancer patients, the prerequisite for an ideal cancer adjuvant differ from conventional adjuvants for several reasons. First, the patients that will receive the vaccines are immuno-compromised because of - for example - impaired mechanisms of antigen presentation, non-responsiveness of activated T cells and enhanced inhibition by regulatory T cells. Second, the tumor antigens are usually self-derived and therefore poorly immunogenic. Third, tumors develop escape mechanisms to avoid the recognition by the immune system, such as tumor editing, low or non-expression of MHC class I molecules or secretion of suppressive cytokines. Thus, adjuvants for cancer vaccines have to be more potent than for prophylactic vaccines (such as used e.g. against infectious diseases) and consequently may be more toxic and may even induce autoimmune reactions. In summary, the ideal cancer adjuvant should rescue and increase the immune response against tumors in immuno-compromised patients, with acceptable profiles of toxicity and safety. Furthermore, the setback with pure recombinant or synthetic antigens used in modern day vaccines is that they are generally far less immunogenic than older style live or killed whole organism vaccines. This has created a major need for improved and more powerful adjuvants for use in these vaccines.

With a few exceptions, alum remains the sole adjuvant approved for human use in the majority of countries worldwide. Although alum is able to induce a good antibody (Th2) response, it has little capacity to stimulate cellular (Th1) immune responses which seem to have particular importance in controlling cancer. In addition, alum has the potential to cause significant local and systemic side-effects including sterile abscesses, eosinophilia and myofascitis, although serious side-effects are relatively rare. In summary, there is a major unmet need for more effective adjuvants suitable for human use. In particular, there is demand for safe and non-toxic adjuvants able to stimulate both, cellular (Th1) immunity as well as humoral immune responses.

The Concept of Therapeutic Cancer Vaccination

The idea of controlling cancer by stimulation of the immune system is not new – initial vaccination strategies to treat cancer patients using Coley's toxin (Nauts 1953) indicated that the immune system can be stimulated in a way that enables to efficiently control tumor growth or - in some cases - even to lyse an existing solid tumor. Apparently, the strong immune response induced by the highly immunogenic bacterial cell wall components caused a systemic inflammation including the release of cytokines, and a multivalent immune response could also have cross-reacted with the tumor. These historic findings demonstrated that the immune system is able to attack tumor cells if recognized (and therefore being immunogenic).

In this context, one hypothesis trying to explain the relatively low frequency of tumor occurrence in immuno-competent hosts is based on the assumption that the immune system is able to eliminate or control the majority of tumors early in their development. Gene mutations acquired during tumor development and expression of neo-antigens or overexpression of cellular proteins can be targets for recognition by the immune system. The hypothesis of immune surveillance – originally developed by Burnet (Burnet 1970) - is supported by clinical data showing that infiltration of tumors by lymphocytes correlate with improved survival for a variety of solid tumor types (Zhang 2003; Nakano 2001; Naito 1998; Schumacher 2001). Also, the high incidence of malignancies in patients receiving chronic immunosuppressive therapy after organ transplantation (Sanchez 2002; Tenderich 2001) as well as the high incidence of lymphomas and Kaposi's sarcomas in patients with HIV-1 infection and AIDS (Goedert 1998) suggests in particular a role of T cell mediated immune mechanisms in immune surveillance of cancer.

However, in contrast to the majority of vaccines existing for infectious agents – where "prophylactic" vaccination is aiming to generate protection against a later exposure of the agent - cancer vaccination has to be performed in a therapeutic setting that attempts to mount an immune response against antigens expressed by the tumor to which the immune system has already been exposed. Therefore, cancer is often associated with an increasingly impaired immune response against the tumor. Escape mechanisms of the tumor such as loss of antigen expression (Marincola 2000), reduced MHC expression (Travers 1982), absence of co-stimulatory molecules (Ochsenbein 2001), suppression of anti-tumor immune responses by $CD4^+CD25^+$ T regulatory (Treg) cells (Antony 2005), and alterations in the cytokine profile (Yamamura 1993) - often skewed towards a Th2 response (Clerici 1998, Rayman 2004) - affect the ability of the immune system to mount an effective response against the growing tumor. In spite of these tumor induced inhibitory mechanisms, there is accumulating experimental evidence indicating that tumor associated antigens (TAA's) can be recognized by T-cells or antibodies resulting in tumor cell destruction (Van der Bruggen 1991, Kawakami 1994, Watson 1996). On the basis of their expression pattern two groups of TAA's can be distinguished: TAA's encoded by mutated cellular genes and TAA's encoded by regular cellular genes. The group of potential TAA's includes mutated tumor suppressor genes, such as p53, mutated oncogene encoded proteins (such as *ras*), mutated cell cycle regulators (CDC27, CDK4) and tumor specific rearrangements of immunoglobulin heavy chain locus (idiotype of B cell neoplasias. TAA's further include *(i)* oncofetal antigens, such as carcinoembryonic antigen (CEA), α-fetoprotein, or human chorionic gonadotropin (hCG), *(ii)* differentiation antigens, such as prostate specific antigen (PSA), melanocyte differentiation antigens (MART-1, tyrosinase, gp100, THP-1, THP-2), *(iii)* overexpressed self antigens (Her2/neu, EpCam [epithelial-cell adhesion molecule], gastrin, and telomerase), and *(iv)* reactivated embryonic gene products ("cancer testes antigens") including MAGE family, BAGE, GAGE and NY-ESO-1. Furthermore, viral gene products, including EBV (Burkitt's nasopharyngeal cancer), HPV (cervical cancer), and HBV (hepatocellular cancer) can serve as targets for immune mechanism. Also, cell surface exposed carbohydrate and mucin antigens resulting from aberrant glycosylation of tumor cells (Mucin-1, SialylTn, Tn, TF, Lewis Y) have been identified in animal models (Fung 1990, Singhal 1991, Zhang S 1997) as susceptible targets for immune therapy. Furthermore, prolonged survival of cancer patients with natural or vaccine-induced antibodies against carbohydrates such as GM2 and SialylTn has been reported (Zhang H 1998, Livingston 1994, MacLean 1996). For example, SialylTn is expressed in more than 80% of cancers of breast, colorectal, prostate and ovarian origin - in contrast to no or very limited expression on the corresponding normal tissues (Itzkowitz 1989, Zhang S 1997, Zhang S 1995) – and correlates with a more aggressive phenotype and poor prognosis (Itzkowitz 1990, Werther 1994).

However, the heterogeneous expression of TAA's on cancer cells makes it necessary to target more than one antigen for eradication of all tumor cells therefore minimizing the risk of escape variants.

The Mechanisms of Cancer Vaccination

Regarding the underlying immunological mechanisms, both, humoral responses with antibodies recognizing surface antigens and T cell responses have been postulated as essential effector mechanisms for eradication of tumor cells. In particular T cells, because of their ability to recognize processed peptides derived from either intracellular or cell membrane antigens, have the potential to recognize altered TAA's.

The initiation of an immune response is a complex process: the processed antigen has to be presented by professional antigen presenting cells in the context with MHC molecules (peptide–MHC complex; 'signal 1') together with the appropriate immune activating signals (costimulatory molecules; 'signal 2') which in turn are usually triggered by a danger signals (Matzinger 2002). Tumor cells, however, do usually not express costimulatory molecules and are unable to prime T cells, and the tumor antigens need to be presented by professional APCs. Dendritic cells (DCs) are the most potent type of APCs that can activate naive T cells and play an important role in the induction of an immune response (Banchereau 1998, Belardelli 2002). DCs are able to deliver exogenous antigens (e.g. derived from lysed tumor cells or protein-based vaccines) into the MHC class II processing pathway to activate helper T cells, and can present endogenous antigens (e.g. derived from viral vector-based vaccines) by

MHC class I molecules to CD8$^+$ T cells. DCs are also capable of delivering exogenous antigens into the MHC class I processing pathway to activate CD8$^+$ T cells (cross-presentation and cross-priming) (Heath 2001, Werdelin 2002). DCs stimulate both the innate and adaptive immune system and have the ability to interact with CD4$^+$ and CD8$^+$ T cells, NK cells and NKT cells.

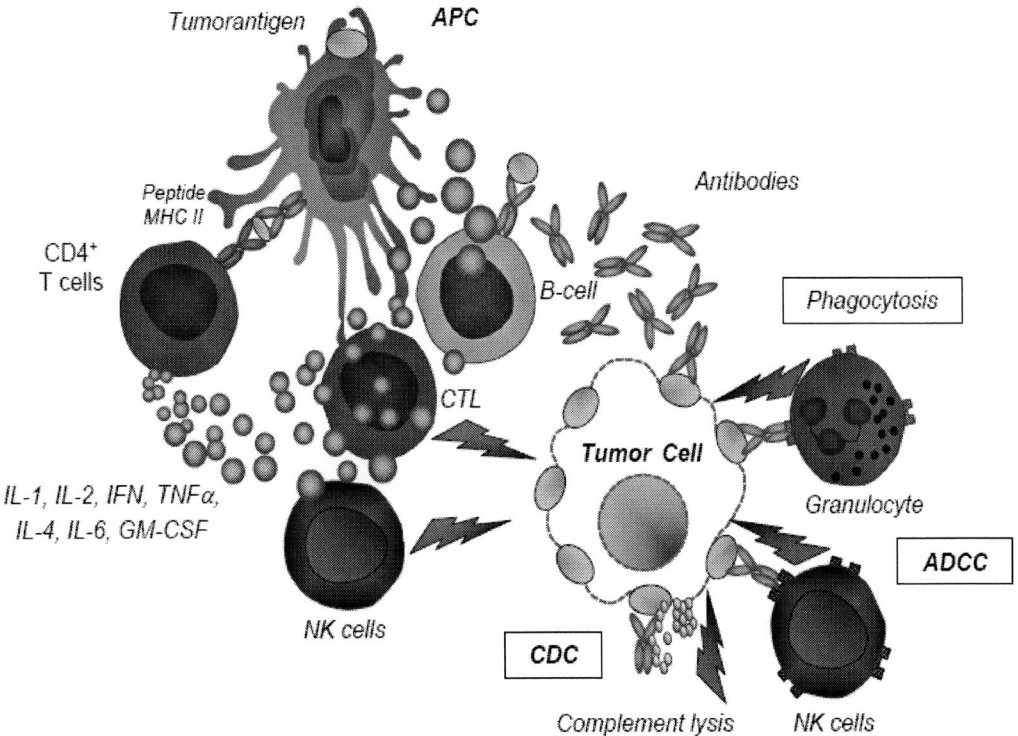

Figure 1: Cellular interactions during induction and effector phases of immune reaction. Following uptake of TAA, the antigen presenting cells (APC, e.g. DC) migrate to the draining lymph nodes where epitopes of the TAA are presented in the context of MHC complex and costimulatory molecules to cognate CD4+ T cells as well as CD8+ T cells. Cytokines released during this interaction contribute to clonal expansion of T cells and B cells. Tumor specific CTLs migrate then to the sites of tumor metastases where they kill tumor cells by perforin mediated cell lysis or apoptosis. CD4+ T cells produced Th1 cytokines may stimulate effector cells of the innate immune system, such as macrophages, NK (natural killer) and NKT cells, which may exert direct anti-tumor effects. Additionally, several Th1 cytokines, such as TNFα and IFNγ, may also excert anti-proliferative or pro-apoptotic effects directly on tumor cells. Th2 cytokines activate B cells producing tumor-specific antibodies, which mediate tumor cell destruction by effector cells via antibody-enhanced mechanisms such as phagocytosis or antibody-dependent cellular cytotoxicity (ADCC), and complement-dependent cytotoxicity (CDC).

The cytokine milieu accompanying this interaction may direct the immune response towards immunity or tolerance (Banchereau 1998). Type-1 cytokines (IL-2, IL-12, IL-15, IFNγ, TNFα and TNFβ) are involved in T helper 1 (Th1) immune responses, primarily inducing cell-mediated immunity. In contrast, type-2 cytokines (IL-4, IL-5, IL-6, IL-10 and

IL-13) are associated with a Th2 immune response promoting humoral immunity (Belardelli F 2002, Dredge 2002).

The initiation of the immune response occurs in the lymph nodes which drain the site of the vaccination (Figure 1). DC's play the critical role in transporting the antigen from the immunization site to the draining lymph node and in presenting and activating naïve antigen specific T cells. DC's are present in immature form throughout the skin and mucosal tissues. Immature DC's are highly effective in capture and uptake of antigens by receptor-mediated endocytosis, pinocytosis, and phagocytosis (Ochsenbein 2001). Following the uptake of antigen and in the presence of stimulatory signals, the DC migrates to the draining lymph nodes via the afferent lymph vessels. During migration, the antigen is processed and the DC undergoes a maturation process, resulting in mature DC that is highly efficient in presenting antigenic peptides to T cells. The mature DC activates the T cells by providing costimulatory signals and they can direct their differentiation into appropriate effector T cells. Mature DC's up-regulate co-stimulatory molecules, such as B7, and present TAA-derived peptides (13–25 mer) to cognate $CD4^+$ T cells in the context of MHC class II molecules. Additional co-stimulatory signals, such as CD40–CD40L interactions further promote DC maturation providing help for efficient priming and activation of $CD8^+$ T cells. DC's can also present 8–11 mer peptides derived from endogenous antigens (e.g. viral vector encoded TAAs) or exogenous antigens (e.g. cross-presentation of recombinant protein vaccine) in the context of MHC class I molecule to $CD8^+$ T cells. $CD4^+$ T cells producing Th1 cytokines, such as IL-2, further contribute to the clonal expansion of $CD8^+$ T cells. Tumor-specific CD8+ T cells migrate to the sites of tumor metastasis where they encounter peptide–MHC complexes presenting the tumor antigen on tumor cells. Cytotoxic T cells (CTLs) are able to kill tumor cells by perforin-mediated cell lysis or by apoptosis mediated through granzymes or death receptor signaling through the Fas-FasL pathway. CTLs secreting IFNγ and TNFα (or TNFβ) may elicit direct or indirect cytotoxic activity. Activated $CD4^+$ T cells may also kill tumor cells by using similar pathways as CTLs. $CD4^+$ T cells producing Th1 cytokines may stimulate effector cells of the innate immune system, such as macrophages, NK (natural killer) and NKT cells, which might exert anti-tumor effects by several mechanisms. Additionally, several Th1 cytokines, such as TNFα and IFNγ, may also exert anti-proliferative or pro-apoptotic effects directly on tumor cells. $CD4^+$ T cells secreting Th2 cytokines are capable of attracting and activating eosinophils resulting in the release of their cytocidal granule content. Th2 cells may also activate B cells producing tumor-specific antibodies, which may contribute to tumor cell destruction by antibody-dependent cellular cytotoxicity (ADCC) and complement-dependent cytotoxicity (CDC). Furthermore, antibodies may also induce an idiotypic (Id) network cascade or tumor-cell apoptosis (for review see Mosolits 2005).

However, when the immune system encounters a new antigen, the outcome is not necessarily activation. Numerous data demonstrate that encounter of antigens by mature T cells often results in the induction of tolerance because of ignorance, anergy or physical deletion (Ohashi 1989; Burkly 1989). What determines the outcome of antigen encounter is the context in which the antigen is presented to the immune system. Thus, the outcome of inflammation or tissue destruction that occurs during viral or bacterial infection (or when the antigen is presented together with the appropriate adjuvant) typically is activation of the immune cascade. In contrast, when the antigen is expressed endogenously - in the absence of the danger signals that typically accompany tissue destruction and inflammation - the typical outcome is immunological tolerance. The underlying principal is that the activation of the T cells is dependent on appropriate costimulatory signals present at the time of antigen recognition. In response to certain danger signals, such as agonists to Toll-like receptors (TLR) or inflammatory cytokines, APCs like Dendritic cells, express the necessary costimulatory molecules such as B7, which promote T cell activation. In the absence of the appropriate costimulatory signals, engagement of the T cell receptor itself typically leads to ignorance, anergy or apoptosis of the antigen specific T cell. Furthermore, carbohydrate antigens are typically much less immunogenic than proteins and generally lack any T cell activating epitopes.

Successful cancer vaccines have to activate both the cellular and humoral arm of the innate and adaptive immune systems (Belardelli 2002). Accumulating data indicate that induction of $CD8^+$ cytotoxic T cells (CTLs) and a Th1-biased CD4+ T cell response are crucial for an efficient anti-tumor response (Gilboa 2004). Additionally, antibodies may be essential in controlling residual disseminated tumor cells in the blood or tissues (Livingston 1994, MacLean 1996, Zhang H 1998).

Adjuvant/ Vaccine Composition

Appropriate adjuvants are supposed to provide the necessary milieu and optimal conditions for effective processing and presentation of the antigen by the ACPs and T cell activation. In particular, the antigen formulation and the cytokine balance have been determined as pivotal factors for effective activation. While soluble antigens often prove to be inferior for effective immunization, particulate formulations have been found to facilitate targeting to antigen presenting cells and efficient uptake into APCs. In addition, the prolonged exposure of the antigen has been found to increase immunogenicity of the antigen formulation. Incorporation of danger signals into antigen formulation – resembling inflammatory responses or tissue destruction – can induce the appropriate cytokine milieu for effective activation of the immune system. Therefore effective adjuvants will have to provide at least three major characteristics to the antigen formulation:

1) Generation of particulate antigen formulation to facilitate uptake into APCs.
2) Formation of a repository or depot of antigen in the tissues to provide a prolonged exposure of the antigen at the APCs
3) Delivery or induction of an appropriate cytokine milieu

Consequently, effective adjuvants should recruit and activate professional APCs and/or immune effector cells, help to deliver antigens to the cytosol and facilitate subsequent cross-priming by mimicking a danger signal (Dredge 2002, Tartour 2002). Preferably, a cancer vaccine adjuvant should promote a Th1-type response (Dredge 2002). The challenge is to develop adjuvants that are effective, yet do not elicit too vigorous immune responses either systemically or at the site of injection, leading to sequelae such as granuloma formation.

Commonly Used Adjuvants

One of the most commonly used adjuvant, aluminium-based salts (alum), acts as a depot formulation and promotes a Th2-polarised immune response (Brewer 1999). Incomplete Freund's adjuvant (IFA) does not seem to be a powerful adjuvant in humans. In contrast, cytokines, particularly GM-CSF (granulocyte-macrophage colony-stimulating factor), have been shown to augment both humoral and cellular immunity by multiple mechanisms of action and facilitate cross-presentation (Mellstedt 1999, Arina 2002). Bacterial DNA containing unmethylated CpG oligodeoxynucleotides is another powerful adjuvant via binding to TLR (Klinman 2003). Products of micro organisms, such as lipopolysaccharide (LPS), Newcastle-disease virus (NDV) and Bacillus Calmette–Guerin (BCG) also exert adjuvant activity probably by providing excessive danger signals. Another examples of adjuvants being evaluated include derivatives of bacterial cell wall component such as monophosphoryl lipid A, Ribi adjuvant, ENHANZYN, microfluidized emulsion of oil and surfactants, e.g. MF59 or SAF-1 (an oil-based emulsion containing muramyl dipeptide and non-ionic block polymer), saponin derivatives, such as QS-21, cationic peptides (poly-arginine, IC31), and polymers such as poly-lactic-poly-glycolic acid.

Ex vivo expanded DCs pulsed with tumor antigens are powerful immunogens. Biodegradable microspheres, virus-like particles, heat-shock proteins (HSPs), and various oil- or lipid-based chemical adjuvants (such as liposomes, ISCOMs, QS-21 or AF) promote cross-presentation of the antigen. Attenuated viral vectors also belong to this category. Helper peptide epitopes (e.g. tetanus toxoid) may also be useful in enhancing and skewing immunity towards a Th1 response (Dredge 2002, Tartour 2002) and may be crucial in inducing immune responses against carbohydrate epitopes.

Delivery systems that might lead to prolonged or pulsative release of the antigen are also under intensive evaluation in order to reduce the number of immunizations required or to boost or to prolong immune responses. Such sustained delivery systems include liposomes or microcapsules composed of biodegradable polymers, such as poly-L-lactide co-glycolide (PLGA) surrounding the antigen. Protection of antigen from rapid degradation, localization of the antigen at the tissue site and providing particles of appropriate size nm till μm for efficient uptake into APC are the major advantages of such formulations. Alternatively, bacterial toxins (such as cholera toxin (CT) or *E. coli* heat-labile toxin (LT) have been used as danger signals to induce appropriate stimulatory cytokines (Tamura 1994). Moreover, cytokines as proteins or in slow release formulations, or secreted by gene-modified tumor cells have been broadly used as adjuvants.

The following section gives an overview on the most commonly used adjuvants as well as some recent developments. While aluminum salts remain the most widely used immunomodulators for human vaccines, a wide variety of agents are being tested to improve the adjuvant properties in various settings and to minimize the potential for side effects. Particular progress has been made in manufacturing processes, the use of large mammals and primates to study mechanisms of action, clinical trials that include validated assays and sufficient power and robust sample size to answer the study objectives, and the management of toxicity by alteration of formulations. Several immunological issues must still be addressed for many adjuvants, such as tolerance, autoimmunity, and immuno-potentiation.

Table 1. Novel adjuvants currently in/close to human clinical testing (adapted from Kenney 2002)

Adjuvant	Brief description	Selected antigen(s)	Source/ supplier	Safety/immunogenicity/ comments
Material salts				
Aluminum or calcium	Aluminum hydroxid and aluminum or calcium phosphate particles	Numerous viral, bacterial and cancer antigens	Superfos, Reheis, others	The predominant adjuvant in current use to provide safe and effective vaccines
Oil emulsion and surfactant-based formulations				
MF59	Microfluidized detergent stabilized oil-in-water emulsion	Influenza, HIVgp120, HSVgD, HBsAg	Chiron	Component of a licensed influenza vaccine in Europe
QS-21	Purified saponin	SPf66, HIVgp120, melanoma	Aquila	Safety profile improved with mixtures
AS02 (SBAS2)	Oil in water emulsion +MPL+QS-21	RTS,S, HIVgp120, SL, L2B7, TRAP	SmithKline Beecham	Reactogenicity acceptable, tolerated in human trials
Montanide ISA-51	Stabilized water in oil emulsion	LSA1/3, SALSA, STARP	Air Liquid Seppic	Slow release properties like IFA
Particulate immunomodulators				
Virosomes	Unilamellar liposomal verhicles with H1N1 influenza A/Singapore	HepA, HepB, influenza vaccine A/A/B	Berna Biotech	i.n. route for influenza is immunogenic with good protection
AS04 (SBAS4)	Al salt with MPL	HBsAg, HSVgD, etc.	SmithKline Beecham	Reactivity acceptable tolerated in human trials
ISCOMS	Structured complex of saponins and lipids	Influenza, HPV16 (E6/E7)	CSL	Slight increase in mild/mod AE over vaccine, well tolerated
Microbial (natural and synthetic) derivatives				

Table 1. (Continued)

Adjuvant	Brief description	Selected antigen(s)	Source/ supplier	Safety/immunogenicity/ comments
Detox (MPL+CWS)	MPL+M. phlei cell wall skeleton	Cancer antigens	Corixa	Approved for use in Canada as a component of Melancine a melanoma vaccine
MPL Adjuvant	Monophosphoryl lipid A	Microbial and cancer antigens	Corixa	Well tolerated in human trials
DC-Chol	Lipoidal immunostimulators able to self organize into liposomes	Influenza, H. pylori urease	Aventis	Parental and intranasal potential
OM-174	Lipid A derivative	PfCS 282-283	OM Pharma	Well tolerated by i.m. route in limited trials
CpG-ODN	Synthetic oligonucleotides containing immunostimulatory CpG motifs	HBsAg, flu (split)	Coley Pharmaceutical group	Mild increase in frequency but not severity of AEs, marked improvements in immunogenicity, species specific sequences
Modified LT and CT	Genetically modified bacterial toxins to provide non-toxic adjuvant effect	H. pylori, pneumo conjugates, RSV	Chiron	Potential for oral and intranasal adjuvant use
Cytokines				
GM-CSF	Plasmid encoded cytokine to augment DNA vaccine responses	PfCSP, EXP-1, LSA1, LSA3, SSP3	Vical	
IL-12	Protein or plasmid encoded cytokine that stimulates Th1	HepA, HepB, pneumo, leish	Genetics Institute	Dose-dependent toxicity

This is particularly true as products begin to be studied in children. This report will summarize the various presentations and is organized by adjuvant type as summarized in Table 1.

Mineral Salts

1. Aluminum Salts

Aluminium adjuvants represent the first adjuvants approved for human use. This group of adjuvants, popularly designated as 'alum', comprises adjuvants such as aluminum hydroxide, aluminum phosphate, and other metal salts, and are currently widely used in a variety of human vaccines. The biologic activity consist of at least three components including (i) formation of a repository or depot of antigen in the tissues to provide a prolonged exposure of the antigen at the antigen presenting site, *(ii)* the generation of particulate antigens to facilitate uptake into APCs, and *(iii)* activation of macrophages and other cells to release cytokine. A slow release of alum-precipitated antigens from the injection site – that is expected to result in prolonged exposure of the immune system to the vaccine antigen resulting in an increased immune response - is dependent on the physical characteristics such as the isoelectric point (pI) of the protein and the aluminium adjuvant, the pH in the tissue and other factors such as presence of phosphate and serum proteins. Interaction of aluminium adjuvant with components of interstitial fluid including phosphate ions, citrate and proteins can lead to rapid desorption of precipitated antigens. As a second mechanism, aluminium gel particles are up to several μm in diameter and can be more efficiently taken up in APCs by phagocytosis than soluble antigens (Ramesh 2007). Alternatively, direct activation of APCs by aluminium adjuvants may result in more efficient uptake also of the desorbed antigen. Aluminum hydroxide was shown to increase the expression of MHC class II molecules and several costimulatory molecules on peripheral blood monocytes accompanied by increased mRNA expression of IL-4, IL-1, TNFα and IL-6 (Ulanova 2001).

Aluminum hydroxide has been used as adjuvant for the cancer vaccine IGN101 with the mAb17-1A adsorbed on aluminium hydroxide. The formulation has been tested in several Phase I and Phase II clinical trials, and was found to be safe in cancer patients (Loibner 2004). The EpCAM binding murine monoclonal antibody mAb17-1A (Riethmüller 1994) which itself contains EpCAM mimicking structures may elicit anti-idiotypic antibodies *in vivo* (Samonigg 1999). The induced anti-idiotypic antibodies might in turn evoke an anti-anti-idiotypic response against the *bona fide* antigen (Fagerberg 1995). The vaccination induced antibodies against EpCAM were reported to show a relationship to a significant reduction of circulating EpCAM positive cells in the peripheral blood. Interim analysis showed that immune responders survived significantly longer than non-responders (Loibner 2004).

The main drawbacks of aluminium adjuvants, however, are their weak or absent adjuvant effect with certain candidate vaccine antigens, the tendency to induce IgE mediated immune responses, and the inability to induce significant cell-mediated and cytotoxic T cell responses. These facts make alum less promising for cancer vaccination where a certain degree of pre-existing tolerance of the host regarding its tumor has to be overcome (Gupta 1998). On the other hand, aluminium adjuvants may serve as a very promising particulate carrier onto which antigens and other, stronger adjuvants with a high potency for T cell activation can be co-formulated. In a recent study, the *per se* non-immunogenic carbohydrate tumor associated antigen SialylTn has been coupled to mAb17-1A, which was used as a highly immunogenic carrier protein (Fagerberg 1993), and formulated onto aluminum hydroxide (Kircheis 2005). Application of this vaccine formulation (designated IGN402) to Rhesus monkeys generated a strong immune response against the xenogenic carrier protein but only a moderate IgM immune response against the SialylTn carbohydrate antigen. However, co-formulation of the vaccine additionally with a strong adjuvant, QS-21, dramatically enhanced the anti-SialylTn immune response and resulted in production of SialylTn-specific IgG antibodies (Kircheis 2006). The induction of carbohydrate-specific IgG antibodies implicates the involvement of carrier-induced T-cell help against the per se T-cell independent carbohydrate antigen. Also a cytokine pattern indicative for induction of a Th1 response was observed (Kircheis 2007).

2. Calcium Phosphate Adjuvant

Calcium phosphate is a commercially available vaccine adjuvant that can potentiate the immune response to antigens. Although its name suggests that it is $Ca_3(PO_4)_2$, X-ray diffraction analysis, FTIR spectroscopy, thermal analysis and the Ca/P molar ratio identify commercial calcium phosphate adjuvant as non-stoichiometric hydroxyapatite, $Ca_{10-x}(HPO_4)_x(PO_4)_{6-x}(OH)_{2-x}$ where x varies from 0 to 2. The surface charge is pH-dependent (isoelectric point = 5.5). Consequently, commercial calcium phosphate adjuvant exhibits a negative surface charge at physiological pH and electrostatically adsorbs positively charged antigens. The presence of hydroxyl groups allows calcium phosphate adjuvant to adsorb phosphorylated antigens by ligand exchange with surface hydroxyls (Jiang 2004).

In murine models, a nanoparticulate adjuvant composed of calcium phosphate was compared to aluminum adjuvants regarding its ability to induce immunity to herpes simplex virus type 2 (HSV-2) and Epstein-Barr virus (EBV) infections. Results indicated that CAP (i) was more potent than alum, (ii) elicited little or no inflammation at the site of administration, (iii) induced high titers of immunoglobulin G2a (IgG2a) antibody and neutralizing antibody, and (iv) facilitated a high percentage of protection against HSV-2 infection. Additional benefits of CAP include (i) a reduced IgE response, which is an important advantage over injection of alum compounds, and (ii) the fact that CAP is a natural constituent of the human body (Gupta 1995). Thus, CAP is very well tolerated and absorbed (He 2000). Regarding testing in clinical studies, diphtheria and tetanus antibody levels were measured before and four weeks after booster vaccination of 313 Danish military recruits participating in a clinical trial to compare aluminium hydroxide and calcium phosphate as adjuvants in diphtheria-tetanus vaccines (DT). The calcium phosphate adsorbed vaccine showed the highest efficacy for both antigens. Adverse reactions were rare but more frequent in the calcium group than in the aluminium group. The results show that calcium phosphate is more effective but not a safer alternative to aluminium hydroxide when compared in vaccines containing 1.0 mg/ml of Ca or of Al (Aggerbeck 1995).

Oil Emulsion and Surfactant-Based Formulations

1. MF59

The squalene based oil-in-water microfluidized emulsion MF59 is the most widely used example of this group that is mainly tested in a variety of influenza vaccines, and has been described as a well tolerated, stable, and metabolizable adjuvant. Incorporation of MF59 was shown to increase immunogenicity of various influenza vaccines (Heineman 1999). Cellular immunity has been augmented by MF59 in murine models leading to the potentiation of IFNγ, IL-4, and IL-2, and it also restores the ability to produce IFNγ that is lost during aging in mice. It has also been shown to induce the production of cytotoxic T lymphocytes (CTL) in monkey models (Heineman 1999, Kenney 2002).

Aluminum hydroxide (alum) and the oil-in-water emulsion MF59 were compared regarding their effects on human immune cells and both were found to induce secretion of chemokines, such as CCL2 (MCP-1), CCL3 (MIP-1α), CCL4 (MIP-1β), and CXCL8 (IL-8) which are all involved in cell recruitment from blood into peripheral tissue. Whereas alum appeared to act mainly on macrophages and monocytes, MF59 was shown to additionally target granulocytes. Accordingly, monocytes and granulocytes migrate toward MF59-conditioned culture supernatants. In monocytes, both adjuvants lead to increased endocytosis, enhanced surface expression of MHC class II and CD86, and down-regulation of the monocyte marker CD14, which are all phenotypic changes consistent with a differentiation toward Dendritic cells (DCs). In addition, MF59 was found to induce further up-regulation of the maturation marker CD83 and the lymph node-homing receptor CCR7 on differentiating monocytes. The studies indicated that during vaccination, MF59 may increase recruitment of immune cells into the injection site, accelerate and enhance monocyte differentiation into DCs, augment Ag uptake, and facilitate migration of DCs into tissue-draining lymph nodes to prime adaptive immune responses (Seubert 2008). Regarding immunization studies in cancer application no clear cut data for efficacy of MF59 have been reported (Asai 2000).

2. QS-21

QS-21 is a purified immunological adjuvant derived from a natural plant source, the bark of the tree *Quillaja saponaria* that is being developed by Aquila Biopharmaceuticals (Framingham, MA, USA) and developed by Antigenics (New York, NY, USA). QS-21 is a water soluble triterpene glycoside with amphiphilic character that can be mixed with a soluble antigen resulting in a fully soluble vaccine formulation or combined with emulsion or mineral salt adjuvants. QS-21 has been shown to enhance antibody, augmented both Th1 and Th2 cytokines, and induced CTL activity cell-mediated immune responses to subunit antigens, as well as DNA vaccines in animal models at microgram doses. It acts as an immunostimulatory adjuvant, eliciting production of immunomodulatory cytokines, and not as an antigen depot. QS-21 is currently under clinical evaluation with various vaccines. This includes a Phase II evaluation of a QS-21 adjuvanted pneumococcal polysaccharide vaccine and a Phase III evaluation of a QS-21 adjuvanted GM2-KLH (ganglioside GM2 vaccine) immunotherapeutic product for melanoma (Kensil 1998).

Therefore, QS-21 is one of the most promising new adjuvants for immune response potentiation and dose-sparing in vaccine therapy given its exceedingly high level of potency and its favorable toxicity profile. Melanoma, breast cancer, small cell lung cancer, prostate cancer, HIV-1, and malaria are among the numerous indications targeted in more than 80 recent and ongoing clinical studies (Kensil 1998).

The generation of the semisynthetic QS-21A(api) adjuvant has been described, applying novel glycosylation methodologies to a convergent construction of the potent saponin immunostimulant. The chemical synthesis of QS-21 offers unique opportunities to probe its mode of biological action through the preparation of otherwise unattainable non-natural saponin analogues (Kim 2006, Wang 2005).

3. GPI-0100

GPI-0100 is a semi-synthetic saponin with modifications designed to augment stability and diminish toxicity. GPI-0100 was tested with doses ranging between 0.1 and 5 mg in groups of five treated prostate cancer patients who had no evidence of disease except for rising PSA levels. GPI-0100 was mixed with a bivalent vaccine containing the glycolipid Globo H and the glycosylated mucin MUC2 conjugated to keyhole limpet hemocyanin (KLH). All doses were well tolerated and antibody titers against Globo H and MUC-2 escalated with the increasing dose levels. At the 5 mg dose level, toxicity remained minimal with only occasional grade II local toxicity at vaccination sites and occasional sporadic grade I elevations in ALT. Compared with a subsequent trial with the same bivalent vaccine plus QS-21 at the maximal tolerated dose of 0.1 mg, the 5 mg dose of GPI-0100 produced comparable antibody titers (Slovin 2005).

4. Water and Oil Emulsions

Montanide adjuvants are either water-in-oil or oil-in-water emulsions. ISA-51 is a water-in-oil emulsion equivalent to IFA and is characterized by slow release of proteins. ISA-720 is similar to an oil-in-water emulsion with rapid release of proteins. An oil-in-water surfactant is able to interact with APC membranes and cause the micro-diffusion of droplets to the draining lymph nodes. Safety studies have shown local reactions with granuloma and abscess formation related to the oil origin (Aucouturier 2000). Non-mineral oil diffuses and gets metabolized causing weak and transitory inflammation as opposed to mineral oils that stay at the injection site and cause strong persistent inflammation. The lengths of the fatty acid chains are important: small chains have solubilizing and detergent-like properties, while long chains are regarded as safe. Toxicity is related to the quality of both, the antigen and the surfactant. Currently ISA-51 (mineral oil based) and ISA-720 (non-mineral oil based) are tested in clinical trials.

Particulate Immunomodulators

1. Virosomes

Virosomes are immunopotentiating influenza virus-like particles built on liposomes composed of 140 nm spherical unilamellar vesicles with influenza H1N1 membrane proteins intercalated in 70% phosphocholine (lecithin), 20% phosphoethanolamine (kephalin) using a detergent technique for formation. The influenza hemagglutinin antigen (HA) binds to sialic acid residues to provide receptor mediated endocytosis and fusion of the virosome with endosomes (Zurbriggen 1999). In humans, the HA antigen is recognized as a highly conserved T cell epitope and is a B cell superstimulatory antigen. Endosomal fusion is part of the MHC class II pathway, which provides for long-lasting immunogenicity with lower reactivity. In combination with *E.coli* heat-labile toxin (LT) the virosomal antigen delivery system can be used for mucosal immunization.

2. ISCOMS

ISCOMs have received much attention as vaccine adjuvants due to their immunostimulatory effects. They are colloidal particles typically comprised of phospholipids, cholesterol and Quil A, a crude mixture of saponins extracted from the bark of *Quillaja saponaria Molina*. ISCOMs can be prepared by ether injection wherein an ether solution of phospholipids and cholesterol is injected into a solution of Quil A. ISCOMs have been prepared from the isolated fractions with four of the fractions identified as QS-7, QS-17, QS-18 and QS-21 (Pham 2006). The ISCOMS formulation ISCOPREP703 has been tested with viral, bacterial, parasitic or cancer antigens by parenteral, intranasal, or oral application routes. A broad range of adjuvant properties is mediated due to targeting of lymphoid organs resulting in a balanced response, with up-regulation of APCs, strong induction of CTLs and antibodies. For adjuvant activity the correct ratio of saponin (QH) to cholesterol and to lipid is a critical parameter (Sjolander 2001). There was limited, short-lived non-specific toxicity and pro-inflammatory changes in high doses and moderate increases in local and systemic reactions, but no serious adverse events (SAEs) observed. The association between antigen and particle is critical for delivery to APC resulting in strong cell-mediated cytokine responses and CTLs induction.

Microbial (Natural and Synthetic) Derivatives

1. BCG

Application of the bacillus Calmette-Guérin (BCG) is regarded as the most successful immunotherapy against superficial bladder carcinoma recurrences to date. It has shown its efficacy - that is based on complex and long lasting immune activation - and advantage over classical therapeutic strategies. The initial step is the binding of mycobacteria to the urothelial lining, which depends on the interaction of a fibronectin attachment protein on the bacteria surface with fibronectin in the bladder wall. Granulocytes and other immunocompetent mononuclear cells are attracted to the bladder wall and a cascade of proinflammatory cytokines sustains the immune response. In the bladder wall a largely Th1 based cytokine milieu and granuloma-like cellular foci are established. Within this scenario, the most important effector mechanisms might be the direct anti-tumor activity of interferons and the cytotoxic activity of NK cells. Current treatment consists of an induction phase of 6 weeks and a maintenance dose schedule of 3 weeks every three months up to 36. The majority of patients present adverse events related to dose administration due to bladder inflammatory response and on only a few occasions there are major complications like granulomatous prostatitis. Among all the neoplasms tested, only in superficial bladder cancer BCG has been shown to be effective (Vázquez-Lavista 2007).

Several randomised controlled therapeutic vaccine trials in GI malignancies were based on using autologous tumor cells mixed with BCG as adjuvant (OncoVAX) used for vaccination of stage II/III colorectal carcinoma patients after surgery and compared to surgery alone. A total of more than 700 patients were enrolled (Hoover 1993, Harris 2000, Vermorken 1999). Recurrence-free survival was significantly improved in vaccinated patients (Hanna 2001). A positive effect was only seen in colon cancer (Hoover 1993) and was more pronounced in patients with stage II as compared to stage III (Vermorken 1999, Hanna 2001) - patients that received additional booster vaccine doses seemed to do better. The magnitude of the delayed-type hypersensitivity (DTH) response against autologous tumor cells correlated significantly with an improved prognosis (Harris 2000).

A multicenter, randomized controlled phase III clinical trial was performed in stages II and III colon cancer patients with active specific immunotherapy using autologous tumor cells with the bacillus Callmette-Guerin (BCG) vaccine (OncoVAX) in an adjuvant setting. In this study, patients were randomized to receive either OncoVAX therapy or no therapy after surgical resection of the primary tumor. Treatment was stratified by the stage of disease. The results of the study verified that the use of OncoVAX for patients with stage II colon cancer has significant prognostic benefit and a positive clinical outcome (Uyl-de Groot 2005).

2. Lipid A derivatives

The lipid A derivative OM-174, which retains the diglucosamine diphosphate backbone of lipid A with only three lipids, has chemically attenuated toxicity. Chemically, it has a purity of > 96%, is soluble in water, and is stable for 5 years at 4°C (Brandenburg 2000). Protection has been demonstrated in an influenza model, and when used with HBsAg, it stimulates both IgG1 and IgG2a antibodies with induction of CTL. In a therapeutic peritoneal cancer model, anti-cancer activity has been shown with markedly improved survival and cure. A Phase I study to define the maximum tolerated dose (MTD) in cancer patients using OM-174 alone showed that > 1 mg can be administered *i.v.* without inducing unacceptable toxicity. In a clinical Phase I study using OM-174 as an adjuvant, mild local pain was seen, but no systemic adverse events were experienced.

3. MPL Adjuvant, Detox–B (ENHANZYN™)

Monophosphoryl lipid A, MPL, adjuvant is derived from the lipopolysaccharide of *Salmonella minnesota*, contains six fatty acids (Baldridge 1999) and like LPS is thought to target Toll-like receptors. MPL is being studied in numerous late-stage clinical trials with microbial and cancer antigens. A safety profile for MPL has evolved from clinical trials that are similar to that established for alum.

Another adjuvant, Detox–B™ is a combination of MPL and CWS (*M. phlei* cell wall skeleton). It has been approved for use in Canada as a component of Corixa's Melacine melanoma vaccine. Detox–B (now also called ENHANZYN) has been extensively used as part of the Theratope synthetic carbohydrate vaccine developed by Biomira and Merck KoAG (see below).

4. AS02

AS02 (formerly known as SBAS2) is a proprietary emulsion containing MPL and QS-21 that causes strong antibody responses along with Th1 and CTLs. This adjuvant has been tested clinically in tuberculosis (TB), hepatitis B, cancer, malaria, and HIV. Side effects include systemic chills, myalgia, headaches and local pain. Strong preclinical efficacy was found in a TB aerosol challenge model in guinea pigs where nearly as much protection was seen with AS02 (90%) as with Bacillus Calmette-Guérin (BCG, 100%). AS02 has also been studied with human papilloma virus (HPV)-induced genital warts in a Phase II therapeutic study comparing three doses (30, 100, and 300 µg) of the L2E7 antigen given *i.m.* at 0, 2, 4 weeks. A strong antibody boost response was observed after the second injection. Both lymphoproliferation and the IFNγ response were highest in the lowest dose group (for review see Kenney 2002).

In a phase I/II study, patients with solid metastatic MAGE-3-positive tumors (mainly melanoma) were vaccinated with recombinant MAGE-3 protein combined with the immunologic adjuvant AS02B comprised of MPL and QS-21 in an oil-in-water emulsion. The recombinant MAGE-3 protein was made up of a partial sequence of the protein D (ProtD) antigen of *Haemophilus influenzae* fused to the MAGE-3 sequence. The vaccine was given *i.m.* at 3-week intervals. Patients whose tumors stabilized or regressed after 4 vaccinations received 2 additional vaccinations at 6-week intervals. MAGE-3 and ProtD antibody and cellular immune responses were monitored after vaccination. Ninety-six percent (23/24) of the patients vaccinated with MAGE-3 protein in AS02B adjuvant elicited a significant anti-MAGE-3 IgG antibody response after 4 vaccinations, and all developed anti-ProtD IgG antibodies. In 30% of the evaluable patients the IFNγ production was increased in response to MAGE-3. In 37% and 43% of the patients, respectively, IFNγ or IL-5 production was increased in response to ProtD. It is concluded that vaccination of advanced cancer patients with MAGE-3 self-antigen in AS02B adjuvant is able to elicit MAGE-3 specific antibody and a T cell response (Vantomme 2004).

In another study, fifty-seven patients with MAGE-3 positive measurable metastatic cancer, most of them with melanoma, were vaccinated with escalating doses of a recombinant

MAGE-3 protein combined with a fixed dose of the immunological adjuvant SBAS-2, which contained MPL and QS-21. The immunisation schedule included 4 *i.m.* injections at 3-week period intervals. Patients whose disease stabilised or regressed after 4 vaccinations received 2 additional vaccinations at 6-week intervals. The vaccine was generally well tolerated. Among the 33 melanoma patients who were evaluable for tumor response, 2 partial responses, 2 mixed responses and 1 stabilisation were reported. Time to progression in these 5 patients varied from 4 to 29 months (Marchand 2003).

5. CpG Oligodeoxynucleotides

Bacterial DNA sequences are recognized as danger signal by the human immune system. The dinucleotide CG frequency is randomly distributed in bacteria and contains unmethylated cytosines, which are mostly methylated in viral and vertebrate DNA. Vertebrate toll-like receptors (TLRs) sense invading pathogens by recognizing bacterial and viral structures and, as a result, activate innate and adaptive immune responses. Ten human functional TLRs have been reported so far; three of these (TLR7, 8, and 9) are expressed in intracellular compartments and respond to single-stranded nucleic acids as natural ligands. The pathogen structure selectively recognized by TLR9 in bacterial or viral DNA was identified to be CpG dinucleotides in specific sequence contexts (CpG motifs). Short phosphorothioate-stabilized oligodeoxynucleotides (ODNs) containing such motifs are used as synthetic TLR9 agonists, and different classes of ODN TLR9 agonists have been identified with distinct immune modulatory profiles. The TLR9-mediated activation of the vertebrate immune system suggests using such TLR9 agonists as effective vaccine adjuvants for infectious disease, and for the treatment of cancer and asthma/allergy. Immune activation by CpG ODNs has been demonstrated to be beneficial in animal models as a vaccine adjuvant and for the treatment of a variety of viral, bacterial, and parasitic diseases.

Optimized short oligodeoxynucleotides (ODN) – designated CpG ODN – have been shown to induce production of IL-12 and IFNγ which subsequently stimulate IFNγ release in a Th1 bias. In murine studies, alum induces only IgG1 whereas CpG ODN together with alum result in mixed response that is augmented by a second dose (Seeber 1991). CpG oligonucleotides work well as mucosal adjuvants (MUCADJ) to induce the production of IgG and mucosal IgA. Using CpG ODNs which have been selected to stimulate all humans, it was found that 50 μg to 1 mg is an effective dose in hypo-responder orangutans being vaccinated against hepatitis B. Human safety studies have been conducted using CpG ODNs with Engerix-B in an *i.m.* injection at 0, 1, and 6 months.

Anti-tumor activity of CpG ODNs has also been established in numerous mouse models. In clinical vaccine trials in healthy human volunteers or in immunocompromised HIV-infected patients, CpG ODNs strongly enhanced vaccination efficiency. Most encouraging results in the treatment of cancers have come from human phase I and II clinical trials using CpG ODNs as a tumor vaccine adjuvant, monotherapy, or in combination with chemotherapy (for review see Jurk 2007).

6. IC31

The adjuvant IC31, consisting of a vehicle based on the anti-microbial cationic peptide KLKL(5)KLK and an immunostimulatory oligodeoxynucleotide containing deoxy-Inosine/deoxy-Cytosine (ODN1a), was found to promote efficient Th1 immune responses mediated via the TLR9/MyD88-dependent pathway of the innate immune system. In mice, IC31 induces potent peptide-specific type 1 cellular immune responses, as well as a mainly type 1 dominated protein-specific cellular and humoral immune responses. In addition, cytotoxic T lymphocytes were induced, able to kill efficiently target cells in vivo. Activation of murine Dendritic cells by IC31 induced efficiently proliferation of naïve $CD4^+$ TCR transgenic T cells as well as their differentiation into IFNγ and IL-4 producing T cells in vitro (Schellack 2006.)

7. Bacterial Toxins

Studies on the mechanism of toxins of enteric bacteria have led to investigation of bacterial toxins as adjuvants (Tamura 1994; Glenn 1998). These include *E.coli* heat-labile toxin (LT) or cholera toxin (CT) as well as tetanus toxoid. Another bacterial toxoid, diphtheria toxoid has extensively been used in cancer immunization studies with the anti-gastrin vaccine (Anti-gastrin 17 immunogen, G17DT, Gastrimmune) developed by Aphton. Gastrin 17 is a growth factor for pancreatic, stomach and colorectal cancers, and a potent stimulator of gastric acid secretion. The anti-gastrin immunogen, G17DT, consisted of a large carrier protein, Diptheria Toxoid (DT) and a synthetic peptide, which is similar to a portion of the gastrin 17 hormone (GT), attached to the carrier protein. These are then contained in a liquid suspension vehicle. When administered to patients, G17DT induces an immune response producing antibodies, which cross-react and neutralise the target hormone thus preventing its interaction with disease-causing or -participating cells. A Phase III, multicenter, double-blind, randomized, controlled trial of G17DT versus placebo in patients with advanced pancreatic cancer confirmed improved survival of patients in the G17DT group through an intention-to-treat analysis. However, the results of a randomized, double-blind, multinational, multicenter study of G17DT in combination with gemcitabine versus placebo and gemcitabine in patients with advanced pancreatic cancer failed to show improved overall survival except on subset analysis of patients with high antibody titers (Gilliam 2007).

8. Heat Shock Proteins

Heat shock proteins have been the focus of many experimental studies during the last few years in order to understand their biology and their immunologic features. Hsp's are natural biological adjuvants that have shown potential in cancer vaccination were hsp gp96 (of the endoplasmic reticulum) and hsp70 (in the cytosol) act as immunological adjuvants (Udono 1994, Przepiorka 1998). These hsp's, or chaperonins, have the capacity to bind a wide array of peptides. Immunization with either native gp96 or hsp70 purified from tumor cells (which carry arrays of tumor-specific peptides) generate systemic anti-tumor immunity (Tamura 1997). The capacity of certain hsp's to act as adjuvants is based upon two features. First, the peptide-loaded gp96 has been shown *in vitro* to effectively introduce antigens into the MHC class I processing pathway as well as into the MHC class II pathway of APCs. Second there is evidence that binding of gp96 to macrophages induces the secretion of pro-inflammatory cytokines. The group of Parmiani et al (2006) conducted clinical studies of vaccination using hsp gp96 purified from autologous tumor tissues in patients with melanoma and colorectal carcinoma. The results of these trials in metastatic melanoma patients with measurable disease showed that a melanoma-specific T cell response can be generated or increased in approximately 50% of vaccinated patients. Moreover, signs of clinical responses were obtained consisting of two complete responses and three long-lasting disease stabilizations. Similar results were obtained in patients with liver metastases of colorectal cancer made disease-free by surgery. In both studies a clear association was found between T cell immune response induced by the vaccine and clinical response both in the trial of melanoma (tumor response) and in that of colorectal cancer patients (disease-free and overall survival at 5 years).

Vaccination with tumor-derived heat-shock protein gp96 induced *in vivo* expansion of MHC class I restricted IFNγ producing T cells recognizing colorectal carcinoma, cells, which was related to improved disease-free and overall survival (Mazzaferro 2003).

Cytokines as Adjuvants

Cytokines regulate both, the cells of the innate immune system (like NK cells, macrophages, and neutrophils) and the adaptive immune system - the T and B cell immune responses. They can act either locally or at a distance and can either enhance or suppress immunity. Two cytokines, IL-2 and IFNγ have been approved by the FDA for treatment of a variety of cancer indications.

1. Interferon Alpha 2b (IFNα-2b)

Two recombinant IFNα products, IFNα-2a and IFNα-2b, are commercially available. Indications in FDA-approved labeling for interferon alfa include the treatment of hairy-cell leukemia, acquired immunodeficiency syndrome-related Kaposi's sarcoma, and genital warts. However, it also is being used successfully against early chronic myelogenous leukemia, low-grade non-Hodgkin's lymphoma, cutaneous T-cell lymphoma, and previously untreated multiple myeloma. Other malignancies that respond to treatment with interferon alfa are malignant melanoma, ovarian carcinoma, and renal cell carcinoma. The toxicity pattern of interferon alfa consists of flu-like symptoms, which are seen at all doses, on all schedules, and in virtually all patients. After repeated dosing anorexia, weight loss, and malaise and fatigue may develop. Myelosuppression, central nervous system toxicity, increased hepatic enzyme concentrations, nausea and vomiting, and cardiovascular toxicity also are possible.

Serum neutralizing antibodies may be formed during therapy - this phenomenon may affect the clinical outcome (Koeller 1989, Marotta 2006). Recently a pegylated IFNα-2b with improved pharmacokinetic parameters has been tested in a variety of clinical cancer indications. The final results of EORTC 18991, a randomised phase III trial with adjuvant therapy with pegylated IFNα-2b in resected stage III melanoma have recently been reported in Lancet. 1256 patients with resected stage III melanoma were randomly assigned to observation (n=629) or pegylated IFNα-2b (n=627) 6 μg/kg per week for 8 weeks (induction) then 3 μg/kg per week (maintenance) for an intended duration of 5 years. The primary endpoint was recurrence-free survival. The median length of treatment with pegylated IFNα-2b was 12 months. The data showed that adjuvant pegylated IFNα-2b for stage III melanoma has a significant, sustained effect on recurrence-free survival (Eggermont 2008).

2. Interleukin 2 (IL-2)

IL-2 is a central cytokine essential for cell growth and activation of T- and B-lymphocytes, activation of natural killer cells as well as macrophages. High doses of IL-2 are being used for generation of lymphokine activated killer (LAK) cells. IL-2 is being used to treat renal cell carcinoma, melanoma, lymphoma, and leukemia. Clinical trials demonstrated that the systemic administration of recombinant high-dose bolus intravenous IL-2 (720 kIU/kg every 8 hours) mediated objective tumor progression in 20% of patients with metastatic renal cancer and in 17% of patients with metastatic melanoma, with complete responses of 9% and 7%, respectively (Rosenberg 2007, Yang 2003, Rosenberg 1994). However, infusion of recombinant IL-2 at those doses which are necessary for therapeutic effects, have been found to often result in significant side effects, such as vascular leakage syndrome (Rosenstein 1986).

3. Interleukin 12 (IL-12)

IL-12 is a heterodimeric cytokine produced by phagocytic cells, professional antigen-presenting cells such as Dendritic cells and skin Langerhans cells, and B cells. IL-12 production is induced by bacteria, intracellular pathogens, fungi, viruses, or their products in a T-cell-independent pathway or a T-cell-dependent pathway, the latter mediated through CD40 ligand-CD40 interaction. IL-12 is produced rapidly after infection and acts as a proinflammatory cytokine eliciting production of interferon gamma, by T and natural killer cells, which activates phagocytic cells. The production of IL-12 is strictly regulated by positive and negative feedback mechanisms. If IL-12 and IL-12 induced IFNγ are present during early T-cell expansion in response to antigen, T-helper type 1 cell generation is favored and generation of T-helper type 2 cells is inhibited. Thus IL-12 is also a potent immunoregulatory cytokine that promotes T-helper type-1 differentiation and is instrumental in the T-helper type 1-dependent resistance to infections by bacteria, intracellular parasites, fungi, and certain viruses by inhibiting T-helper type 2 cell response (Trinchieri 1995). The clinical development of IL-12 as a single agent for systemic cancer therapy has been hindered by its significant toxicity and disappointing anti-tumor effects. The lack of efficacy was accompanied by, and probably related to, the declining biological effects of IL-12 in the course of repeated administrations at doses approaching the maximum tolerated dose (MTD). Nevertheless, IL-12 remains a very promising immunotherapeutic agent because recent cancer vaccination studies in animal models and humans have demonstrated its powerful adjuvant properties (Portielje 2003).

3. GM-CSF (Granulocyte-Macrophage Colony Stimulating Factor)

GM-CSF stimulates the differentiation of hematopoetic progenitors to monocytes and neutrophils, and reduces the risk for febrile neutropenia in cancer patients. GM-CSF also has been shown to induce the differentiation of myeloid dendritic cells (DCs) that promote the development of T-helper type 1 (cellular) immune responses in cognate T cells. GM-CSF has been used to augment the activity of rituximab in patients with follicular lymphoma and to induce autologous antitumor immunity in patients with hormone-refractory prostate cancer. GM-CSF causes the up-regulation of costimulatory molecule expression on leukemia blasts in vitro, enhancing their ability to present antigen to allogeneic T cells, and, in combination with IFNγ, can induce anti-tumor immune responses in patients whose acute leukemia has relapsed following allogeneic hematopoietic progenitor cell transplant. Tumor cells engineered to secrete GM-CSF are particularly effective as anti-tumor vaccines, and the addition of GM-CSF to standard vaccines may increase their effectiveness by recruiting DCs to the site of vaccination (Waller 2007).

This new role for myeloid-acting cytokines in regulating immune responses is also based on their activity on dendritic cell maturation and activation. Subsets of DCs may augment or inhibit cellular immune responses. Enhanced DC1 activity has been associated with enhanced cytotoxic immune responses. Granulocyte-macrophage-colony-stimulating factor (GM-CSF) and granulocyte-colony- stimulating factor (G-CSF) differ by their effects on enhancing the numbers or activity of DC1 or DC2 subsets of DCs, respectively. The increase in DC1 content and activity following local and systemic GM-CSF administration support a role for GM-CSF as an immune stimulant and vaccine adjuvant in cancer patients. The clinical activity of GM-CSF in anti-tumor immune responses has been documented in its use in tumor cell and DC vaccines. Nevertheless, a significant anti-tumor effect of parenterally administered GM-CSF in a randomized clinical study has yet to be consistently demonstrated. The successful use of myeloid acting cytokines to enhance anti-tumor responses will likely require targeting these drugs or activating DCs directly into the tumor microenvironment (Arellano 2004).

Barrio et al (2006) have investigated the adjuvant effect of recombinant hGM-CSF with respect to the immunogenicity of VACCIMEL, a vaccine consisting of 3 irradiated allogeneic melanoma cell lines. A phase I clinical trial was performed in 20 melanoma patients. Cohorts of 4 patients were vaccinated 4 times with VACCIMEL and bacillus Calmette Guerin (BCG) as adjuvant. Additionally, the patients received placebo or GM-CSF at four different doses (150, 300, 400, 600 mg per vaccine). The combination of VACCIMEL and GM-CSF had low toxicity. Delayed-type hypersensitivity increased after vaccination and it was highest in the group with the highest GM-CSF dose (Barrio 2006).

In a phase I clinical trial, eleven end-stage melanoma patients were vaccinated intradermally with 3 peptides: MART-1, tyrosinase, and gp100, mixed with tetanus toxoid and GM-CSF. The peptide vaccine was well tolerated at all tested doses, and led to grade 1-2 toxicity only. Although all patients did show a rise in anti-tetanus IgG titers, in only 3 patients peptide-specific CD8 T cells were induced. However, none of the 11 patients responded clinically according to response evaluation criteria in solid tumors criteria (Bins 2007).

In another clinical Phase I trial twelve radically operated colorectal carcinoma patients were immunized with three injections of ALVAC-KSA - an avipox virus with an inserted full-length EpCAM gene either alone or together with GM-CSF (75 µg/day for four consecutive days). ALVAC-KSA, in combination with low dose local administration of GM-CSF was shown to induce a strong, IFNγ T-cell response (type 1) with high titers of IgG antibodies and a late boosted T cell response (Ullenhag 2003).

Summarizing these studies using a variety of recombinant cytokines administered together with vaccines immunological proof of principle has been multifold demonstrated in a variety of models, however, the clinical response rate of individual cytokines was usually low. Moreover, infusion of cytokines was often found to be associated with significant side effects and in most cases only a modest therapeutic effect has been shown so far (Schiller 1996, Panelli 2004, Kammula 1998). This limited efficacy may be explained by the failure to recapitulate accurately the paracrine and synchronized function of cytokines in the context of antigen uptake and presentation (Pardoll 1995). Furthermore, the synchronized action of a cytokine orchestra rather than single cytokines may be required for optimal induction of an immune response. Studies using combined cytokines in the ratios they are produced naturally have shown that the combinations can have synergistic effects. These combinations of cytokines can also be used to enhance the effects of vaccines designed to stimulate the immune system to mount a cancer cell specific immune response (Kircheis 1998, 2007).

Cytokine therapy can induce tumor regression in cancer patients but systemic administration of cytokines is often accompanied with severe toxicity. Loco-regional delivery may represent a more effective and less toxic alternative to systemic injection. However, the requirement for frequent repeated injections of recombinant cytokine or the logistical difficulties associated with gene-modification have limited wide-spread use of loco-regional therapy.

Paracrine Cytokine Adjuvants

An alternative approach has been explored that produces high concentrations of cytokines in the vicinity of the tumor. This is achieved either by transduction of the tumor cells with the cytokine gene or by mixture of the tumor cells with cytokine containing biodegradable slow release formulations (such as microspheres). Under these circumstances, the locally released cytokine produces a strong local inflammatory response specific to the particular cytokine. In some cases, a potent tumor specific T cell response results, capable of mediating regression of systemic tumor deposits. This paracrine delivery of cytokines can therefore be considered as an important improvement in the design of vaccines for cancer as well as microbial infections.

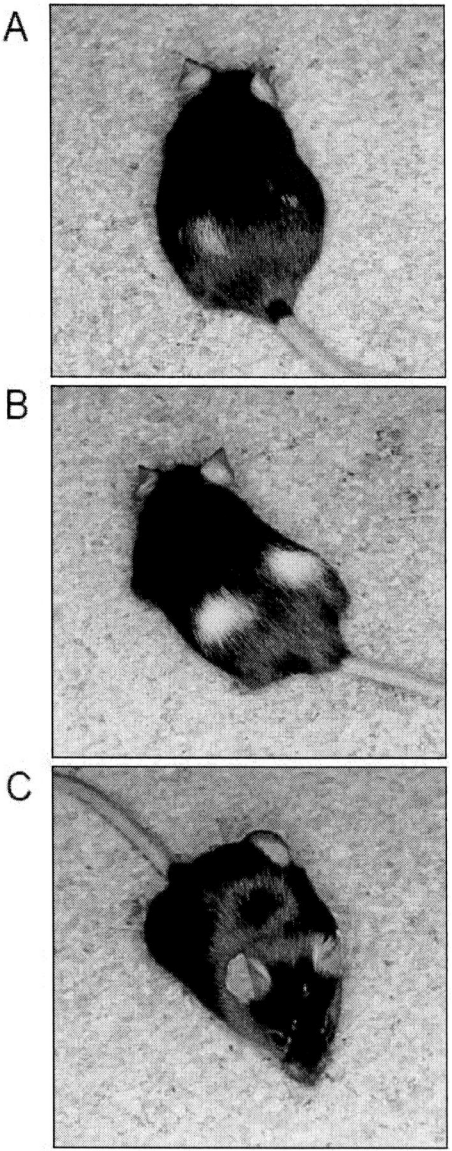

Figure 2. Protection of mice against a lethal challenge with B16 melanoma cells and development of vitiligo after vaccinations with IL-2 liposomes admixed to irradiated tumor cells. C57Bl/6 mice (H-2^b) were vaccinated twice with 2×10^5 irradiated syngeneic B16-F10 cells (24 mice), or with 2×10^5 irradiated syngeneic B16-F10 cells, admixed with liposomes containing IL-2 (22 mice). Release of IL-2 was in 300 ng per 24 hrs. One week after second vaccination all mice were challenged with 1×10^5 wild-type B16-F10 cells. Whereas all animals of the control group developed tumors (C), 11/22 of the vaccinated animals were protected from tumor challenge with several of them developing vitiligo at the vaccination sites (right) and/or tumor challenge site (left) (A,B).

A simple local delivery strategy is the use of controlled-release cytokine depot formulations. These formulations provide the advantage that physiological doses of cytokines are directly released to the tumor microenvironment in a sustained manner. Anti-tumor efficacy of IL-2, IL-12, GM-CSF or TNFα encapsulated polymer microspheres has been evaluated in syngeneic murine and human tumor /SCID mouse xenograft models. A single intra-tumoral injection of these formulations; particularly that of IL-12 in combination with GM-CSF or TNFα was shown to promote the regression of established primary tumors; induced systemic anti-tumor T- and NK cell responses and achieved complete eradication of disseminated disease - these effects were associated with the activation of tumor-associated T effector/memory cells; the elimination of $CD4^+$ $CD25^+$ $Foxp3^+$ T suppressors and the *de novo* priming of tumor-specific $CD8^+$ T effector cells (Egilmez 2007).

In a preclinical study, subcutaneous vaccination of C57Bl/6 mice with irradiated B16 melanoma cells supplemented with liposomal murine IL-2 or murine IFNγ resulted in systemic protection in 50% of the animals, against a subsequent tumor cell challenge in a dose dependent manner (Figure 2). The protective efficacy was comparable to the efficacy of cytokine gene-modified cells as tumor vaccine, whereas irradiated B16 cells supplemented with soluble cytokine did not result in protective responses. Their studies showed that the beneficial effects mediated by liposome incorporation of the cytokine are the result of a depot function of the liposomal cytokine supplement at the vaccination site (van Slooten 1999, Koppenhagen 1998).

In hepatocellular carcinoma (HCC) a tumor cell-based vaccine combined with adjuvant cytokines in slow release formulations significantly improved overall and disease-free survival in a nonrandomized Phase I/II clinical trial compared to resection alone. The HCC vaccine consisted of autologous formalin-fixed tumor tissue fragments, biodegradable microparticles containing human granulocyte macrophage colony-stimulating factor and human IL-2, and tuberculin (Kuang 2004).

1. Cytokine Gene Modified Tumor Cells for Anti-Cancer Vaccination

A widely used delivery strategy is the use of cytokine gene modified tumor cells as source of both, tumor associated antigens and adjuvant. In a variety of animal models the modification of tumor cells with the genes of immunostimulatory cytokines was shown to inhibit the growth of these cells when transplanted into syngeneic hosts (Fearon 1990, Gansbacher 1990b, Colombo 1991). When used as vaccines, cytokine gene-modified tumor cells have been found to induce protection against subsequent challenge with wild-type tumor cells and, in some cases, against pre-existing tumor deposits (Fearon 1990, Gansbacher 1990a ,1990b, Porgador 1993, Zatloukal 1995). Recent data have indicated that local delivery of immunostimulatory cytokines at the site of tumor antigen uptake / processing is crucial for the induction of a systemic antitumor immune response (Golumbek 1993, Pardoll 1995, Jaffee 1996). The efficacy of the induced anti-tumor immune response was found to depend on (i) the parameters of the tumor model, such as tumorigenicity, immunogenicity, tumor load, location, (ii) the cytokine used, (iii) the cytokine dosage, and (vi) immunization scheme such as number of immunizations or the spacial distribution of the vaccine inoculum (Dranoff

1993, Zatloukal 1995, Connor 1993, Schmidt 1995, Jaffee 1996). While certain cytokines, such as GM-CSF seem to act in a dose-response relation which shows saturation at high doses, for other cytokines, such as IL-2, a bell-shaped dose-dependency was found (Schmidt 1995). These data indicate that for maximal efficacy of a cytokine, a therapeutic dose-window has to be defined. The situation gets even more complex when two or more cytokines are co-administered. On the other hand, under certain conditions co-application of different cytokines acting at different steps of the immune cascade may be expected to lead to additive or synergistic effects. In a preclinical study two immunostimulatory cytokines: IL-2 and IFNγ were compared with the combination of both cytokines for their potency as adjuvants in prophylactic and therapeutic vaccination protocols in two syngenic mouse melanoma models. The data indicate that the efficacy of the vaccination is dependent on the tumor load, as well as on the cytokine doses and combination. The combination of both cytokines was found to be superior to the single cytokine treatments (Kircheis 1998).

In multiple murine models, GM-CSF has been shown to be one of the most potent immunostimulatory products. Vaccination with irradiated tumor cells engineered to secrete GM-CSF involves enhanced tumor antigen presentation by recruited dendritic cells (DCs) and macrophages; the coordinated functions of $CD4^+$ and $CD8^+$ T cells, CD1d-restricted NKT cells and antibodies mediate protective immunity. The evaluation of this vaccination strategy in patients with advanced melanoma revealed the consistent induction of cellular and humoral anti-tumor responses capable of effectuating substantial necrosis of distant metastases (Dranoff 2002, 2003).

A phase I clinical trial was performed to test the effect of vaccination with irradiated, autologous melanoma cells engineered to secrete GM-CSF by adenoviral-mediated gene transfer. The average GM-CSF secretion was 745 ng/ 10^6 cells/ 24 hours. Toxicities were restricted to grade 1 to 2 with local skin reactions. Vaccination elicited dense dendritic cell, macrophage, granulocyte, and lymphocyte infiltrates at the injection sites in 19 of 26 assessable patients. Immunization stimulated the development of delayed-type hypersensitivity reactions to irradiated, dissociated, autologous, nontransduced tumor cells in 17 of 25 patients. Metastatic lesions that were resected after vaccination showed brisk or focal T-lymphocyte and plasma cell infiltrates with tumor necrosis in 10 of 16 patients. One complete, one partial, and one mixed response were noted. Ten patients (29%) were alive, with a minimum follow-up of 36 months with four of them having no evidence of disease (Soiffer 2003).

Vaccination with irradiated autologous NSCLC cells engineered to secrete GM-CSF was also found to enhance anti-tumor immunity in some patients with metastatic NSCLC in a phase I clinical trial (Salgia 2003).

2. Cytokine Gene Modified Allogeneic Tumor Cells for Anti-Cancer Vaccination

Cellular vaccines can be divided into autologous - derived from the patient's own tumor - and allogeneic vaccines. Autologous vaccines have the advantage of containing all potentially relevant TAAs of the particular patient. However, autologous vaccines are difficult to obtain from most patients with advanced disease and impossible to obtain from patients who present after tumor. The amount of autologous tumor available is rarely enough to produce more than two or three vaccination doses, and the time between initial tumor harvest and ultimate availability of the vaccine may result in interval tumor progression that diminishes the likelihood of vaccine efficacy. All these drawbacks of autologous tumor vaccination limit its applicability and also limit the ability to test autologous vaccines in prospective trials (Sondak 2006).

An attractive alternative approach is to apply standardized gene-modified tumor cell lines as allogeneic vaccines to a broad variety of patients. This strategy is based on the findings that (*i*) a number of tumor antigens are shared between different tumors (Gaughler 1994, Kawakami 1994, Rodolfo 1991) and (*ii*) priming of $CD4^+$ and $CD8^+$ T cells occurs most probably mainly via professional APCs of the host ('indirect priming') rather than by the tumor cells themselves ('direct priming') making MHC-matching between vaccinating tumor cells and the recipient unnecessary (Pardoll 1995, Huang 1994, Maass 1995). Furthermore, recent studies have shown that expression of an allogeneic MHC molecule (Plautz 1993, Thomas 1998) or admixing of allogeneic GM-CSF gene-modified bystander cells to a syngeneic vaccine (Thomas 1998) do not inhibit the induction of the anti-tumor response but can even improve it, supporting the concept of allogeneic vaccination. Potential advantages offered by the allogeneic approach have led to a variety of preclinical and clinical studies with cytokine-gene-modified, allogeneic melanoma cell lines.

Knight et al. (1996) found some cross-protection against the B16F10 melanoma induced by allogeneic vaccines. Another group showed that the anti-tumor activity was significantly enhanced by modification of the cells with the GM-CSF gene (Kayaga 1999). Kircheis et al (2000) demonstrated that allogeneic vaccination can induce cross-protection against a syngeneic tumor with efficacy comparable to syngeneic vaccines, providing additional support for the hypothesis that MHC matching is not required. Release of immunostimulatory cytokines at the vaccination site is necessary for efficient protection, both for syngeneic and for allogeneic vaccination (Figure 3). The efficacy of allogeneic vaccination, however, was found to depend on maximal sharing of relevant tumor rejection antigens between the vaccinating cells and the recipient and on other characteristics of the patient's tumor.

Regarding efficacy in clinical studies, tumor vaccines composed of autologous tumor cells genetically modified to secrete GM-CSF (GVAX) have demonstrated clinical activity in advanced-stage non-small-cell lung cancer (NSCLC). In an effort to remove the requirement for genetic transduction of individual tumors, a 'bystander' GVAX platform composed of autologous tumor cells mixed with an allogeneic GM-CSF-secreting cell line was tested in a phase I/II trial in advanced-stage NSCLC. Serum GM-CSF pharmacokinetics were consistent with secretion of GM-CSF from vaccine cells for up to 4 days with associated transient leukocytosis confirming the bioactivity of vaccine-secreted GM-CSF. Evidence of vaccine-induced immune activation was demonstrated, however, objective tumor responses were not seen. Compared with autologous GVAX vaccines prepared by transduction of individual tumors with an adenoviral GM-CSF vector, vaccine GM-CSF secretion was approximately 25-fold higher with the bystander GVAX vaccine used in this trial. However, the frequency of vaccine site reactions, tumor response, time to disease progression, and survival were all less favorable in the current study (Nemunaitis 2006).

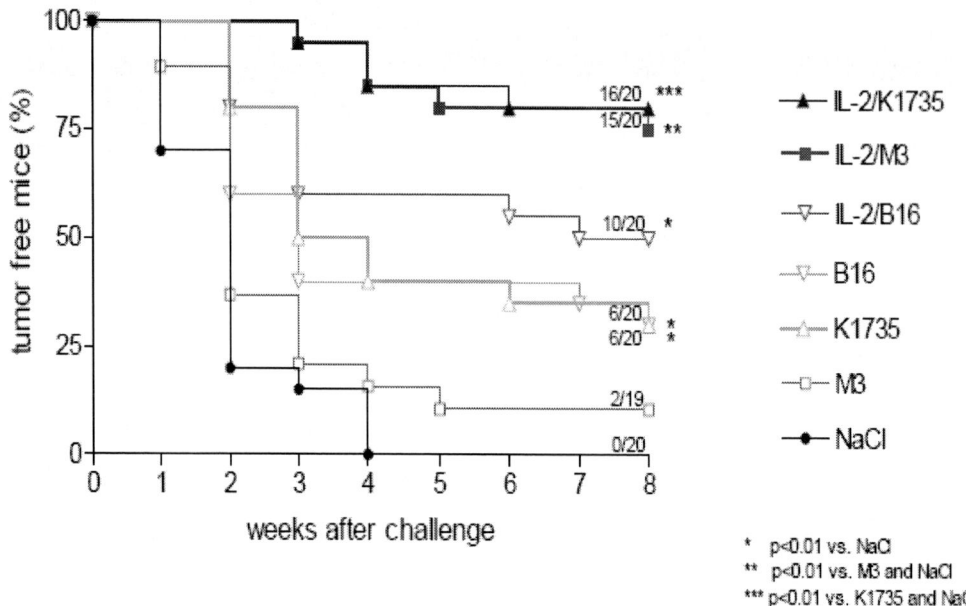

Figure 3: IL-2 gene-transfection increases efficacy of syngeneic and allogeneic vaccination. DBA/2 mice (H-2^d) (20 animals per group) were vaccinated twice with either 1x10^6 IL-2 gene-transfected, irradiated allogeneic B16-F10 cells (H-2^b), IL-2 gene-transfected, irradiated allogeneic K1735 cells (H-2^k), or IL-2 gene-transfected, irradiated syngeneic M-3 cells (H-2^d). Expression of IL-2 was approximately 300 ng per 24 hrs. For comparison, animals were vaccinated with either 1x10^6 non-transfected, irradiated allogeneic B16-F10 or K1735 cells, or non-transfected, irradiated syngeneic M-3 cells. One week after second vaccination mice were challenged with 3x10^5 wild-type M-3 cells. As control, one group of non-vaccinated animals was challenged with the same tumor cell dose. Tumor growth was monitored for eight weeks. Numbers of protected animals are shown. Differences in the development of tumors between different vaccination groups were statistically analyzed using the Logrank test.

Recently a clinical study was performed to determine the safety and feasibility of vaccination with a retrovirally transduced allogeneic prostate carcinoma cell line, LNCaP, expressing IL-2 and IFNγ and to evaluate the efficacy of inducing tumor-specific immune responses in HLA-A2-matched patients with hormone refractory prostate cancer (HRPC). Immunization with the allogeneic LNCaP/ IL-2/ IFNγ vaccine was found to be safe and feasible without any dose-limiting toxicity or autoimmunity.

A 50% PSA decline was achieved in two of the six patients. This encouraging data provides the scientific rationale for further investigation of the vaccine in a phase II trial (Brill 2007).

Synthetic Peptide Cancer Vaccines

Cellular cancer vaccines, while having the potential advantage of having all or the majority of relevant TAAs incorporated, have the disadvantage of being very labor intensive and may have difficulties to meet regulatory requirements and to be reproducibly produced at industrial scale. Therefore synthetic cancer vaccines would be the choice in terms of practicability, regulatory requirements and production. As with cellular vaccines, the incorporation of effective adjuvants is essential to provide sufficient immunogenicity.

Re-activated cancer germline genes, such as genes of the MAGE, BAGE and GAGE families have been identified to encode for TAA's recognized by T-lymphocytes (van der Bruggen 1991, Gaughler 1994). The MAGE-3 antigen presented by HLA-A1 has been used in several vaccination trials on metastatic melanoma patients. Applying this approach, a correlation between tumor regression and anti-MAGE-3.A1 CTL responses in patients vaccinated with a recombinant virus encoding the antigen and also in patients vaccinated with peptide pulsed dendritic cells was found. In contrast, for patients showing tumor regression after vaccination with peptide alone, CTL responses were almost never observed (Lonchay 2004).

In another clinical trial, 24 pretreated patients with relapsed high-risk resected stage IIA-IV melanoma received adjuvant peptide vaccinations derived from the melanosomal antigens MelanA/MART1, MAGE-1, gp100, and tyrosinase, according to patient tumor-associated human leukocyte antigen (HLA) antigen expression, in combination with GM-CSF. All patients received peptide vaccines in an adjuvant setting. Seven patients were relapse free for 3+ up to 25+ months, 17 patients exhibited progressive disease. Vaccine treatment was well tolerated, with no severe side-effects. Twenty out of twenty-four patients developed local delayed-type hypersensitivity (DTH) reactions to synthetic peptide vaccination. Transient fever and pain in muscle/bone occurred rarely. In conclusion, antigenic peptide vaccination, combined with GM-CSF, was found to be safe and may yield clinical benefits in relapsed high-risk resected melanoma patients (Atzpodien 2007).

In another clinical trial twelve peptides derived from melanocyte differentiation proteins and cancer-testis Ags were combined and administered in a single mixture to patients with resected stage IIB, III, or IV melanoma. Three of the peptides (MAGE-A1(96-104), MAGE-A10(254-262), and gp100(614-622)) were found immunogenic when administered with GM-CSF in Montanide ISA-51 adjuvant. T cells secreting IFNγ in response to peptide-pulsed target cells were detected in peripheral blood and in the sentinel immunized node, the node draining a vaccine site, after three weekly injections. The magnitude of response typically reached a maximum after two vaccines, and though sometimes diminished thereafter, those responses typically were still detectable 6 weeks after the last vaccines. Most importantly, tumor cell lines expressing the appropriate HLA-A restriction element and MAGE-A1, MAGE-A10, or gp100 proteins were lysed by corresponding CTL's.

A melanoma vaccine composed of a HLA-A2-restricted peptide derived from gp100(280), with or without a modified T helper epitope from tetanus toxoid, was evaluated in a Phase I trial to assess safety and immunological response. The vaccines were administered s.c. in either of two adjuvants, Montanide ISA-51 or QS-21, to 22 patients with high-risk resected melanoma (stage IIB-IV). Local and systemic toxicities were mild and transient. CTL responses to the gp100(280) peptide were detected in 14% of patients. Helper T-cell responses (Th1) to the tetanus helper peptide were detected in 79% of patients. The overall survival of patients was 75% at 4.7 years follow-up, which compares favorably with expected survival. Data from this trial demonstrated immunogenicity of the gp100(280) peptide and that immune responses may persist long-term in some patients (Slingluff 2001). Because cancer-testis antigens are expressed in multiple types of cancer, MAGE-A derived peptides may be considered for inclusion in vaccines against cancers of other histological types, in addition to melanoma (Chianese-Bullock 2005).

Carbohydrate Antigen Cancer Vaccines

Beside protein and peptide based tumor-associated antigens also TAAs resulting from aberrant glycosylation, e.g. SialylTn, Tn, Lewis Y (LeY) or GloboH, are frequently over-expressed on cancer cells and provide potential targets for cancer vaccination. Cell surface exposed carbohydrate and mucin antigens resulting from aberrant glycosylation of tumor cells have been demonstrated as susceptible targets for immune therapy in animal models (Fung 1990, Singhal 1991, Zhang S 1995, Haurum 1999). Furthermore, prolonged survival of cancer patients with natural or vaccine-induced antibodies against carbohydrates such as GM2 and SialylTn has been reported (Zhang H 1998, Livingston 1994, MacLean 1996). SialylTn is expressed in more than 80% of cancers of breast, colorectal, prostate and ovarian origin, in contrast to no or very limited expression on the corresponding normal tissues (Itzkowitz 1989, Zhang S 1997, Zhang S 1995). SialylTn expression by various epithelial cancers correlates with a more aggressive phenotype and poor prognosis (Itzkowitz 1990, Werther 1994).

While carbohydrates have been recognized as clinically most relevant antigens for vaccine development against infectious diseases, however, in cancer patients, many of the defined carbohydrate antigens represent altered 'self' antigens. Although these self antigens have been found to be potentially suitable targets for immune recognition and killing, the development of vaccines for cancer treatment is actually more challenging compared with those for infectious diseases because of the difficulty associated with breaking the body's immunological tolerance to the antigen. Because these antigens lack the inherent immunogenicity associated with bacterial antigens and, therefore, methods to enhance immunological recognition and induction of immunity *in vivo* are of particular importance. These include defining the appropriate TAAs, successfully synthesizing the antigen to mimic the original molecule, inducing an immune response, and subsequently enhancing the immunological reactivity. This has been successfully accomplished with several glycolipid and glycoprotein antigens using carriers, e.g. keyhole limpet haemocyanin (KLH) together with a saponin adjuvant, QS-21 showing high titre IgM and IgG antibodies, which are specific for the antigen used for immunization, and antibody mediated complement lysis (Slovin 2005).

1. Theratope

Theratope vaccine is a synthetic carbohydrate based cancer vaccine that was designed by Biomira, Inc. (Edmonton, Alberta, Canada) by incorporating a synthetic SialylTn (STn) antigen that emulates the carbohydrate seen on human tumors formulated together with the nonspecific immune stimulants Keyhole Limpet Hemocyanin (KLH) and Detox-B stable emulsion (now called ENHANZYN Immunostimulant). A large number of patients with various adenocarcinomas, including colon cancer have been vaccinated with Theratope (the sialyl-Tn antigen conjugated to keyhole limpet hemocyanin). Patients that developed high IgG titres against mucin sialyl-Tn (STn) epitopes survived longer, and anti-STn IgM titre was shown to be an independent positive prognostic factor for colon cancer (Reddish 1996; MacLean 1996).

Between 1995 and 2000, 70 patients (16 with stage II/III breast cancer, 17 with stage III/IV ovarian cancer, and 37 with stage IV breast cancer) were treated with different formulations of STn-KLH and the observed toxicity, the study outcome, and the immune response data are reported. Generally, STn-KLH was well-tolerated with minimal toxicity and the most common side effects were indurations and erythema at the sites of injections. Humoral and cellular responses were elicited in the majority of the patients. Overall, these data indicate that post-autologous transplant patients are able to mount an effective immune response to vaccine immunotherapy with minimal side effects, and that vaccine immunotherapy may be a useful addition to high-dose chemotherapy regimens (Miles 1996, Miles 2003, Holmberg 2003). Both, in a non-transplant setting following low dose i.v. cyclophosphamide and in the high dose autologous transplant setting, there has been a trend toward Theratope vaccine decreasing the risk for relapse, prolonging the time to relapse and thus impacting on overall survival.

The definitive Phase III trial comparing the outcome of patients with metastatic breast cancer receiving vaccinations with Theratope vaccine versus vaccination included over 1000 women with distant metastatic breast cancer (Holmberg 2001). Whereas very promising results were found in the Phase II trials, the Phase III failed to show statistically significant superiority of the treatment group compared to the control group (Ibrahim 2003).

In a recent study a vaccine based on clustered (instead of single) sTn-KLH [sTn(c)-KLH] conjugate plus QS-21 was tested for immunization of high-risk breast cancer patients. Induction of IgM and IgG antibodies against synthetic sTn(c) and natural sTn on ovine submaxillary mucin were measured before and after therapy. The most common toxicities were transient local skin reactions at the injection site and mild flu-like symptoms. All patients developed significant IgM and IgG antibody titers against sTn(c). Antibody titers against ovine submaxillary mucin were usually of lower titers. IgM reactivity with LSC tumor cells was observed in 21 patients and with MCF-7 cells in 13 patients. There was minimal IgG reactivity with LSC cells. Immunization with sTn(c)-KLH conjugate plus QS-21 is well tolerated and immunogenic in high-risk breast cancer patients. The authors concluded the incorporation of sTn(c) as a component of future multiple antigen vaccines (Gilewski 2007).

2. Multi-Epitope Vaccines

While synthetic carbohydrate cancer vaccines have been shown to induce specific immune responses against immunizing antigen, the heterogeneous expression of TAA's on cancer cells, however, makes it necessary to target more than one antigen for maximal eradication of tumor cells to minimize the risk of escape variants.

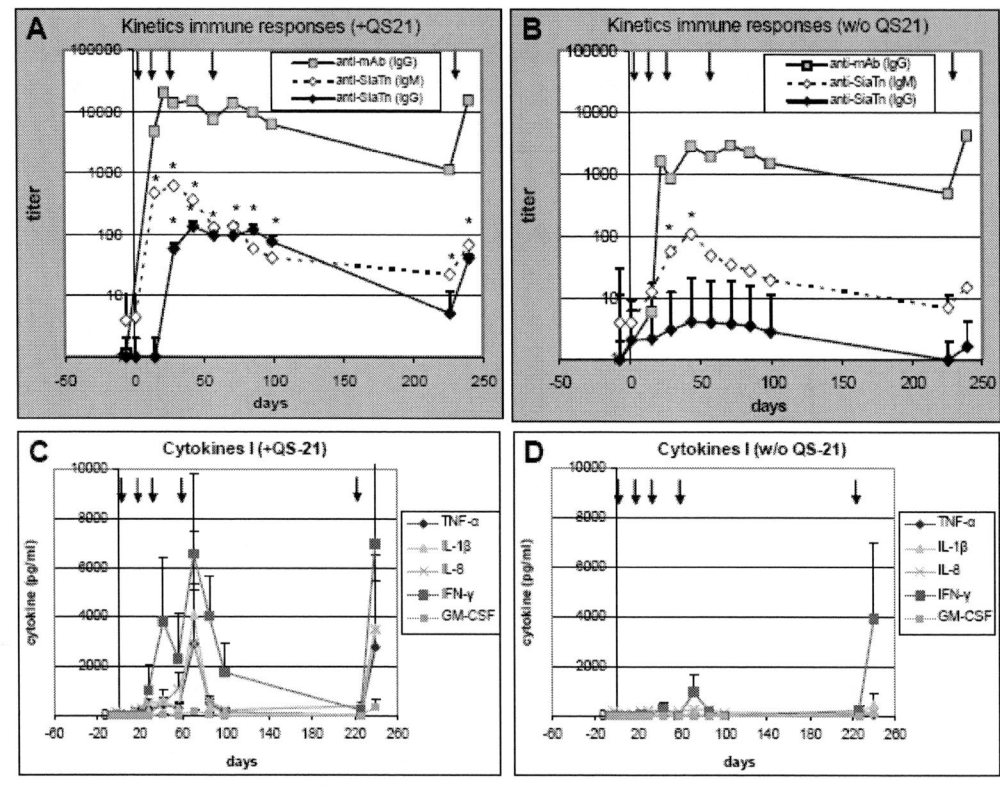

Figure 4. Immune responses against carrier protein and SialylTn and cytokine release after immunization with SialylTn-mAb17-1A vaccine with or without co-formulation with QS-21. Rhesus monkeys (four animals per group) were immunized with SialylTn-mAb17-1A vaccine with (A,C) or without (B,D) QS-21 adjuvant at days 1, 15, 29, 57 and re-boosted at day 226. Pre-sera and immune sera were analyzed for immune response by ELISA. The kinetics of the immune responses, i.e. antibody titers (geomean and scatter factor) against SialylTn (IgG, IgM) and mAb17-1A (IgG) are shown (A, B). Pre-serum and immune sera were analyzed for cytokine release by xMAP technology (Luminex). Cytokine levels (pg/ml) measured in serum are shown (mean and SD) (C, D). Statistics: * $p < 0.05$ vs. Pre-serum (one-tailed, paired t-test).

Combining several target specificities on a single molecule would be pharmaceutically most favorable (Ragupathi 2002, Ragupathi 2003). A variety of multi-epitope cancer vaccine prototypes have been tested so far (Ragupathi 2002, 2006, Slovin 2007, Livingston 2007) with the most advanced among them being a heptavalent antigen-keyhole limpet hemocyanin (KLH) plus QS-21 vaccine construct tested for safety and immunogenicity in patients with epithelial ovarian, fallopian tube, or peritoneal cancer in second or greater complete clinical remission. Eleven patients in this pilot trial received a heptavalent vaccine s.c. containing GM2 (10 mg), Globo-H (10 mg), Lewis Y (10 mg), Tn(c) (3 mg), STn(c) (3 mg), TF(c) (3 mg), and Tn-MUC1 (3 mg) individually conjugated to KLH and mixed with adjuvant QS-21 (100 mg). Vaccinations were administered at weeks 1, 2, 3, 7, and 15. Eleven patients were included in the safety analysis; 9 of 11 patients remained on study for at least 2 weeks past fourth vaccination and were included in the immunologic analysis (two withdrew, disease progression).

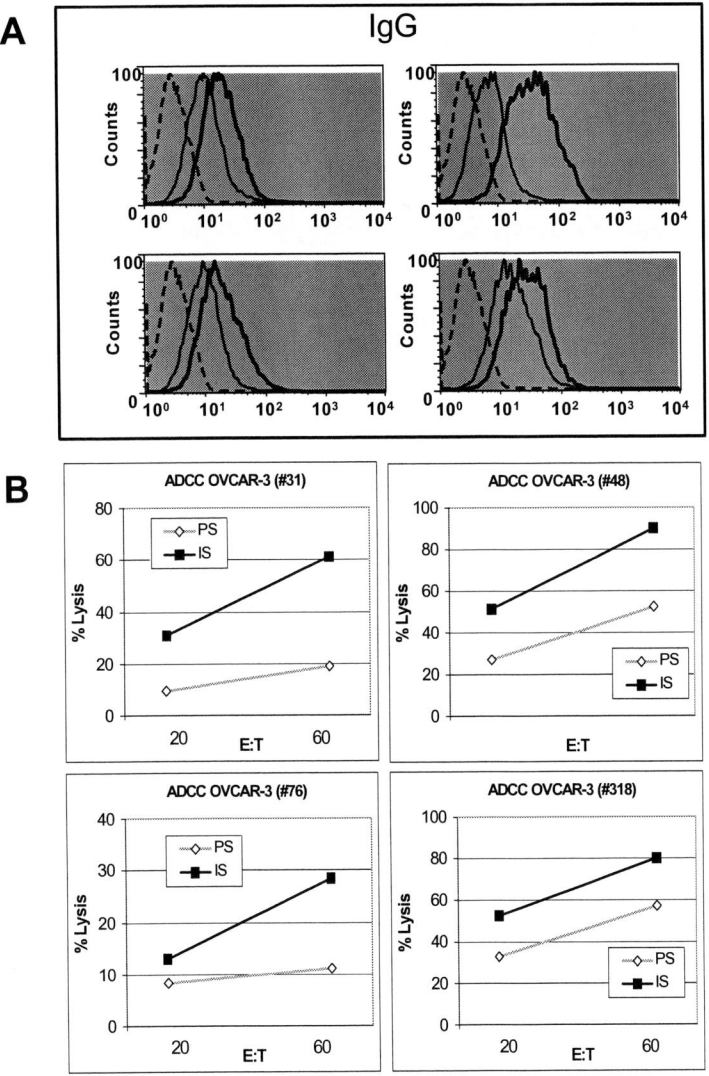

Figure 5. Cell binding to SialylTn positive OVCAR-3 cells and ADCC after immunization with SialylTn-mAb17-1A vaccine co-formulated with QS-21. Rhesus monkeys were immunized with the SialylTn-mAb17-1A vaccines co-formulated with QS-21. Pre-serum and immune sera were analyzed for cell binding (IgG) to SialylTn positive OVCAR-3 tumor cells by FACS analysis (A) and for ADCC activity against SialylTn positive OVCAR-3 cells. Human PBMCs were used as effector cells and incubated with the 51Cr-labeled target cells at E:T ratios of 60:1 and 20:1 for 14h. ^{51}Cr-release was measured using a γ-counter (B).

The vaccine was well tolerated. Self-limited and mild fatigue (maximum grade 2 in two patients), fever, myalgia, and localized injection site reactions were most frequent. No clinically relevant hematologic abnormalities were noted and no clinical or laboratory evidence of autoimmunity was seen. Serologic responses by ELISA were largely IgM against each antigen with the exception of Tn-MUC1 where both IgM and IgG responses were induced. After immunization, median IgM titers were as follows: Tn-MUC1, 1:640 (IgG 1:80); Tn, 1:160; TF, 1:640; Globo-H, 1:40; and STn, 1:80. Only one response was seen against Lewis Y; two were against GM2. Eight out of nine patients developed responses against at least three antigens. Antibody titers peaked at weeks 4 to 8 in all patients. Fluorescence-activated cell sorting and complement-dependent cytotoxicity analysis showed substantially increased reactivity against MCF7 cells in seven of nine patients, with some increase seen in all patients. This heptavalent-KLH conjugate plus QS-21 vaccine safely induced antibody responses against five of seven antigens (Sabbatini 2007).

Another strategy for building multi-epitope vaccines is to couple tumor associated carbohydrate epitopes to a highly immunogenic murine antibody with intrinsic anti-tumor activity in order to (*i*) use an immunogenic carrier protein to increase the immunogenicity of the carbohydrate antigen and to (*ii*) capitalize on the anti-tumor immune response induced by the carrier molecule itself (Fagerberg 1993, Fagerberg 1995, Fagerberg 1996). IGN402 is a first candidate of this type of conjugate vaccines consisting of SialylTn carbohydrate epitopes chemically coupled to mAb17-1A. The murine 17-1A antibody - a monoclonal antibody (mAb) recognizing the epithelial cell adhesion molecule (EpCAM) has been used for passive cancer therapy in patients with epithelial carcinomas (Riethmüller 1994) whereby part of the observed efficacy has been attributed to the induction of anti-idiotypic and anti-anti-idiotypic antibodies (Fagerberg 1993, Fagerberg 1996, Fagerberg 1995). Following these observations the murine 17-1A antibody has been adsorbed on aluminum hydroxide and used as vaccine antigen in the cancer vaccine candidate IGN101, and has been reported to prolong survival in metastatic colorectal cancer patients (Settaf 2004).

In recent studies an immunogenic formulation of SialylTn-mAb17-1A conjugate on alhydrogel (designated IGN402) with or without additional adjuvants was tested in Rhesus monkeys for tolerability and immunogenicity. The conjugate vaccine IGN402 co-formulated with QS-21 adjuvant was found to induce a significant humoral response (IgM and IgG) against the SialylTn carbohydrate antigen and binding reactivity against SialylTn positive tumor cells. A temporary release of cytokines measurable in the serum by xMAP Multiplex technology was induced following repeated immunization. Induction of carbohydrate-specific IgG - requiring T-cell help – was found to correlate with release of pro-inflammatory cytokines including IFNγ, IL-2, IL-1 and GM-CSF (Figure 4). The data demonstrated that coupling of T-cell independent, poorly immunogenic carbohydrates, such as SialylTn, to a murine monoclonal antibody, formulated in the presence of strong adjuvants can dramatically increase immunogenicity and provide carrier-induced T-cell help sufficient for carbohydrate specific antibody IgG class switch induction (Figure 5). Beside the tumor-specific immune response, an increased tumor cell lysis by NK cells, correlating with cytokine release after boost immunization was observed (Figure 4).

In conclusion, these studies indicate that molecularly defined synthetic vaccines eliciting a specific immune response against defined target antigen(s) together with a synchronized cytokine release may be promising candidates for cancer vaccine development.

References

Aggerbeck, H; Fenger, C; Heron, I. Booster vaccination against diphtheria and tetanus in man. Comparison of calcium phosphate and aluminium hydroxide as adjuvants-II. *Vaccine,* 1995; 13(14): 1366-1374.

Antony, PA; Restivo, NP. CD4+CD25+ T regulatory cells, immunotherapy of cancer and interleukin-2. *J. Immunother,* 2005; 28: 120-128.

Arellano, MK; Waller E. Granulocyte-macrophage-colony-stimulating factor and other cytokines: as adjuncts to cancer immunotherapy, stem cell transplantation, and vaccines. *Curr Hematol Rep,* 2004; 3(6):424-431.

Arina, A; Tirapu, I; Alfaro, C; et al. Clinical implications of antigen transfer mechanisms from malignant to dendritic cells, exploiting cross-priming. *Exp Hemato,* 2002; 30: 1355–1364.

Asai, T; Storkus, WJ; Whiteside, TL. Evaluation of the modified ELISPOT assay for gamma interferon production in cancer patients receiving antitumor vaccines. *Clin Diagn Lab Immunol,* 2000; 7(2):145-154.

Atzpodien, J; Reitz, M; GM-CSF plus antigenic peptide vaccination in locally advanced melanoma patients. *Cancer Biother Radiopharm,* 2007; 22(4):551-555.

Aucouturier, J; Ganne, V; Laval, A; Efficacy and safety of new adjuvants. *Ann New York Acad Sci,* 2000; 916: 600–604.

Baldridge, JR; Crane, RT; Monophosphoryl lipid A (MPL) formulations for the next generation of vaccines. *Methods* 1999; 19: 103–107.

Banchereau, J; Steinman, RM; Dendritic cells and the control of immunity. *Nature* 1998; 392: 245–252.

Barrio, MM; de Motta, PT; Kaplan, J; von Euw, EM; Bravo, AI; Chacón, RD; Mordoh, J. A phase I study of an allogeneic cell vaccine (VACCIMEL) with GM-CSF in melanoma patients. *J Immunother.* 2006; 29(4): 444-54

Belardelli, F; Ferrantini, M; Cytokines as a link between innate and adaptive antitumor immunity. *Trends Immunol.* 2002; 23: 201–208

Bins, A; Mallo, H; Sein, J; van den Bogaard, C; Nooijen, W; Vyth-Dreese, F; Nuijen, B; de Gast, GC; Haanen, JB. Phase I clinical study with multiple peptide vaccines in combination with tetanus toxoid and GM-CSF in advanced-stage HLA-A*0201-positive melanoma patients. *J Immunother.* 2007; 30(2): 234-239

Brandenburg, K; Lindner, B; Schromm, A; et al. Physicochemical characteristics of triacyl lipid A partial structure OM-174 in relation to biological activity. *Eur J Biochem.* 2000; 267: 3370–3377.

Brewer, JM; Conacher, M; Hunter, CA; et al. Aluminium hydroxide adjuvant initiates strong antigen-specific Th2 responses in the absence of IL-4- or IL-13-mediated signaling. *J Immunol.* 1999; 163: 6448–6454.

Brill, TH; Kübler, H; von Randenborgh, H; Fend, F; Pohla, H; Breul, J; Hartung, R; Paul, R; Schendel, DJ; Gansbacher, B. Allogeneic retrovirally transduced, IL-2- and IFN-gamma-secreting cancer cell vaccine in patients with hormone refractory prostate cancer--a phase I clinical trial. *Gene Med.* 2007; 9(7): 547-560

Burkly, LC; Lo, D; Kanagawa, O; Brinster, RL; Flavell, RA. *Nature.* 1989; 342: 564-566

Burnet, FM. The concept of immune surveillance. Prog. Exp. *Tumor Res*. 1970; 13: 1-27

Chianese-Bullock, KA; Pressley, J; Garbee, C; Hibbitts, S; Murphy, C; Yamshchikov, G; Petroni, GR; Bissonette, EA; Neese, PY; Grosh, WW; Merrill, P; Fink, R; Woodson, EM; Wiernasz, CJ; Patterson, JW; Slingluff, CL Jr. MAGE-A1-, MAGE-A10-, and gp100-derived peptides are immunogenic when combined with granulocyte-macrophage colony-stimulating factor and montanide ISA-51 adjuvant and administered as part of a multipeptide vaccine for melanoma. *J Immunol*. 2005; 174(5): 3080-3086.

Clerici, M; Shearer, GM; Clerici, E; Cytokine Dysregulation in invasive cervical carcinoma and other human neoplasias: time to consider the Th1/Th2 paradigm. *J. Natl. Cancer Inst*. 1998; 90: 261-263.

Colombo, MP; Ferrari, G; Stoppacciaro, A; et al. Granulocyte colony-stimulating factor gene transfer suppresses tumorigenicity of a murine adenocarcinoma in vivo. *J. Exp. Med. 1991;* 173: 889-897.

Connor, J; Bannerji, R; Saito, S; et al. Regression of bladder tumors in mice treated with interleukin-2 gene-modified tumor cells. *J. Exp. Med.* 1993; 177: 1127-1134.

Dranoff, G. GM-CSF-based cancer vaccines. *Immunol Rev*. 2002; 188: 147-154.

Dranoff, G. GM-CSF-secreting melanoma vaccines. *Oncogene*. 2003; 22(20): 3188-3192

Dranoff, G; Jaffee, E; Lazenby, A; et al. Vaccination with irradiated tumor cells engineered to secrete murine granulocyte-macrophage colony-stimulating factor stimulated potent, specific, and long-lasting anti-tumor immunity. *Proc. Natl Acad. Sci. USA*. 1993 90: 3539-3543.

Dredge, K; Marriott, JB; Todryk, SM; et al. Adjuvants and the promotion of Th1-type cytokines in tumor immunotherapy. *Cancer Immunol Immunother*. 2002; 51: 521–531.

Eggermont, AM; Suciu, S; Santinami, M; Testori, A; Kruit, WH; et al. Adjuvant therapy with pegylated interferon alfa-2b versus observation alone in resected stage III melanoma: final results of EORTC 18991, a randomised phase III trial. *Lancet*. 2008; 372(9633): 117-126.

Egilmez, NK; Kilinc, MO; Gu; T, Conway, TF. Controlled-release particulate cytokine adjuvants for cancer therapy. *Endocr Metab Immune Disord Drug Targets*. 2007; 7(4): 266-270.

Fagerberg, J; Ragnhammar, P; Liljefors, M; Hjelm, AL; Mellstedt, H; Frodin, JE. Humoral anti-idiotypic and anti-anti-idiotypic immune response in cancer patients treated with monoclonal antibody 17-1A. Cancer Immunol. *Immunother*. 1996; 42: 81-87

Fagerberg J, Frodin JE, Wigzell H, Mellstedt H. Induction of an immune network cascade in cancer patients treated with monoclonal antibodies (ab1). I. May induction of ab1-reactive T cells and anti-anti-idiotypic antibodies (ab3) lead to tumor regression after mAb therapy? Cancer Immunol. Immunother. 37: 264-270, 1993.

Fagerberg, J; Hjelm, AL; Ragnhammar, P; et al. Tumor regression in monoclonal antibody-treated patients correlates with the presence of anti-idiotype-reactive T lymphocytes. *Cancer Res* 1995; 55: 1824–1827.

Fearon, ER; Pardoll, DM; Itaya, T; et al, Interleukin-2 production by tumor cells bypasses T helper function in the generation of an antitumor response. *Cell*. 1990; 60: 397-403.

Fung, PYS; Madej, M; Koganty, RR; Longenecker, BM. Active specific immunotherapy of a murine mammary adenocarcinoma using a synthetic tumor-associated glycoconjugate. *Cancer Res.* 1990; 50: 4308-4314.

Gansbacher, B; Bannerji, R; Daniels, B; et al. Retroviral vector-mediated γ-interferon gene transfer into tumor cells generates potent and long-lasting antitumor immunity. *Cancer Res*. 1990; 50: 7820-7825.

Gansbacher, B; Zier, K; Daniels, B; et al. Interleukin-2 gene transfer into tumor cells abrogates tumorigenicity and induces protective immunity. *J. Exp. Med.* 1990b; 172: 1217-1224.

Gaughler, B; Van den Eynde, B; van der Bruggen, P; Romero, P; Gaforio, JJ; DePlaen, E; Lethe, B; Brasseur, F; Boon, T. Human gene MAGE-3 codes for an antigen recognized on a melanoma by autologous cytolytic T lymphocytes. *J. Exp.Med.* 1994; 179: 921-930.

Gilboa, E. The promise of cancer vaccines. Nat. Rev. Cancer. 2004; 4: 401-411.

Golumbek, PT; Azhari, EM; Jaffee, LM; et al. Controlled release, biodegradable cytokine deposits: a new approach in cancer vaccine design. *Cancer Res.* 1993; 53: 5841-5844.

Gilewski, TA; Ragupathi, G; Dickler, M; Powell, S; Bhuta, S; Panageas, K; Koganty, RR; Chin-Eng, J; Hudis, C; Norton, L; Houghton, AN; Livingston, PO. Immunization of high-risk breast cancer patients with clustered sTn-KLH conjugate plus the immunologic adjuvant QS-21. *Clin Cancer Res.* 2007; 13(10):2977-2985.

Gilliam, AD; Watson, SA. G17DT: an antigastrin immunogen for the treatment of gastrointestinal malignancy. Expert Opin Biol Ther. 2007; 7(3):397-404.

Glenn, GM; Rao, M; Matyas, GR; Alving, CR. Skin immunization made possible by cholera toxin. *Nature*. 1998; 391: 851.

Goedert, JJ; Cote, TR; Virgo, P; et al. Spectrum of AIDS-associated malignant disorders. *Lancet*. 1998; 351: 1833-1839.

Gupta, RK. Aluminum compounds as vaccine adjuvants. *Adv. Drug Deliv. Rev*. 1998; 32: 155-172.

Gupta, RK; Rost, BE; Relyveld, E; Siber, GR. Adjuvant properties of aluminum and calcium compounds. *Pharm Biotechnol*. 1995; 6:229-248.

Hanna, MG Jr; Hoover, HC Jr; Vermorken, JB; et al. Adjuvant active specific immunotherapy of stage II and stage III colon cancer with an autologous tumor cell vaccine: first randomized phase III trials show promise. *Vaccine*. 2001; 19: 2576–2582.

Harris, JE; Ryan, L; Hoover, HC Jr; et al. Adjuvant active specific immunotherapy for stage II and III colon cancer with an autologous tumor cell vaccine: Eastern Cooperative Oncology Group Study E5283. *J Clin Oncol* 2000; 18: 148–157.

Haurum, JS; Holer, IB; Arsequell, G; Neisig, A; Valencia, G; Zeuthen, J; Neefjes, J; Elliott, T. Presentation of cytosolic glycosylated peptides by human class I major histocompatibility complex molecules in vivo. *J. Exp. Med*. 1999; 190: 145-150

He, Q; Mitchell, AR; Johnson, SL; Wagner-Bartak, C; Morcol, T; Bell, SJ. Calcium phosphate nanoparticle adjuvant. *Clin Diagn Lab Immunol*. 2000; 7(6):899-903.

Heath, WR; Carbone, FR. Cross-presentation, dendritic cells, tolerance and immunity. *Annu Rev Immunol*. 2001; 19: 47–64.

Heineman, TC; Clements-Mann, ML; Poland, GA; et al. A randomized controlled study in adults of immunogenicity oa novel hepatitis B vaccine containing MF59 adjuvant. *Vaccine* 1999; 17: 2769-2778.

Holmberg, LA; Oparin, DV; Gooley, T; Lilleby, K; Bensinger, W; Reddish, MA; MacLean, GD; Longenecker, BM; Sandmaier, BM. Clinical outcome of breast and ovarian cancer patients treated with high-dose chemotherapy, autologous stem cell rescue and THERATOPE STn-KLH cancer vaccine. *Bone Marrow Transplant.* 2000; 25(12): 1233-1241.

Holmberg, LA; Oparin, DV; Gooley, T; Sandmaier, BM. The role of cancer vaccines following autologous stem cell rescue in breast and ovarian cancer patients: experience with the STn-KLH vaccine (Theratope). *Clin Breast Cancer.* 2003; 3 Suppl 4: S144-1451.

Holmberg, LA; Sandmaier, BM. Theratope vaccine (STn-KLH). *Expert Opin Biol Ther.* 2001; 1(5): 881-891.

Hoover, HC Jr; Brandhorst, JS; Peters, LC; et al. Adjuvant active specific immunotherapy for human colorectal cancer: 6.5-year median follow-up of a phase III prospectively randomized trial. *J Clin Oncol.* 1993; 11: 390–399.

Huang, A.Y.C; Golumbek, P; Ahmadzadeh, M; Jaffee, E; Pardoll, D; Levitsky, H. Role of bone marrow-derived cells in presenting MHC class I-restricted tumor antigens. *Science.* 1994; 264: 961-965.

Ibrahim, NK; Murray,JL. Clinical development of the STn-KLH vaccine (Theratope). Clin Breast Cancer. 2003; 3 Suppl 4: S139-143.

Itzkowitz, SH; Bloom, EJ; Kokal, WA; Modin, G; Hakomori, S; Kim, YS. Sialosyl-Tn: a novel mucin antigen associated with prognosis in colorectal cancer patients. *Cancer* 1990; 66: 1960-1966.

Itzkowitz, SH; Yuan, M; Montgomery, CK; Kjeldsen, T; Takahashi, HK; Bigbee, WL; Kim, YS. Expression of Tn, sialosyl-Tn, and T antigens in human colon cancer. *Cancer Res.* 1989; 49: 197-204.

Jaffee, EM; Thomas, MC; Huang, AYC; et al. Enhanced immune priming with spatial distribution of paracrine cytokine vaccines. *Journal of Immunotherapy.* 1996; 19: 176-183.

Jurk, M; Vollmer, J. Therapeutic applications of synthetic CpG oligodeoxynucleotides as TLR9 agonists for immune modulation. *BioDrugs.* 2007; 21(6): 387-401.

Kayaga, J; Souberbielle, BE; Sheikh, N; Morrow, WJW; Scott-Taylor, T; Vile, R; Dalgleish, AG. Antitumor activity against B16F10 melanoma with a GM-CSF secreting allogeneic tumor cell vaccine. *Gene Ther.* 1999; 6: 1475-1481.

Kammula, US; White, DE; Rosenberg, SA. Trends in the safety of high dose bolus interleukin-2 administration in patients with metastatic cancer. *Cancer.* 1998; 83: 797-805.

Kawakami, Y; Eliyahu, S; Delgado, CH; Robbins, PF; Rivoltini, L; Topalian SL; Miki, T; Rosenberg, SA. Cloning of the gene coding for a shared human melanoma antigen recognized by autologous T cells infiltrating into tumor. *Proc. Natl. Acad. Sci. USA* 1994; 91: 3515-3519.

Kenney, RT; Regina Rabinovich, N; Pichyangkul, S; Price, VL; Engers, HD. 2nd meeting on novel adjuvants currently in/close to human clinical testing. World Health Organization-Organisation Mondiale de la Santé Fondation Mérieux, Annecy, France, 5-7 June 2000. *Vaccine.* 2002; 20(17-18): 2155-2163

Kensil, CR; Kammer, R. QS-21: a water-soluble triterpene glycoside adjuvant. *Expert Opin Investig Drugs.* 1998; 7(9): 1475-1482

Kim, YJ; Wang, P; Navarro-Villalobos, M; Rohde, BD; Derryberry, J; Gin, DY. Synthetic studies of complex immunostimulants from Quillaja saponaria: synthesis of the potent clinical immunoadjuvant QS-21Aapi. *J Am Chem Soc.* 2006; 128(36): 11906-11915.

Kircheis, R; Küpcü, Z; Wallner, G; Rössler, V; Schweighoffer, T; Wagner, E. Interleukin-2 gene-modified allogeneic melanoma cell vaccine can induce cross-protection against syngeneic tumors in mice. *Cancer Gene Ther.* 2000; 7: 870-878.

Kircheis, R; Küpcü, Z; Wallner, G; Wagner, E. Cytokine gene-modified tumor cells for prophylactic and therapeutic vaccination: IL-2, IFNγ, or combination IL-2 + IFNγ. *Cytokines Cell Mol Ther.* 1998; 4: 95-103.

Kircheis, R; Vondru, P; Nechansky, A; Ohler, R; Loibner, H; Himmler, G; Mudde, GC. SialylTn-mAb17-1A carbohydrate-protein conjugate vaccine: effect of coupling density and presentation of SialylTn. *Bioconjug Chem.* 2005; 16(6): 1519-1528.

Kircheis, R; Vondru, P; Zinöcker, I; Häring, D; Nechansky, A; Loibner, H; Mudde, GC. Immunization of Rhesus monkeys with the conjugate vaccine IGN402 induces an IgG immune response against carbohydrate and protein antigens, and cancer cells. *Vaccine.* 2006; 24: 2349-2357.

Kircheis, R; Siegl, P; Grunt, S; Halanek, N; Loibner, H; Mudde, GC; Nechansky, A. Immunization of Rhesus monkeys with a SialylTn-mAb17-1A conjugate vaccine co-formulated with QS-21 induces a temporary systemic cytokine release and NK cytotoxicity against tumor cells. *Cancer Immunol Immunother.* 2007; 56(6): 863-873.

Klinman, DM. CpG DNA as a vaccine adjuvant. *Expert Rev Vaccines* 2003; 2: 305–315.

Knight, B.C; Souberbielle, B.E; Rizzardi, G.P; Ball, S.E; Dalgleish, A.G; Allogeneic murine melanoma cell vaccine: a model for the development of human allogeneic cancer vaccine. *Melanoma Res.* 1996; 6: 1-8.

Koeller, JM. Biologic response modifiers: the interferon alfa experience. *Am J Hosp Pharm.* 1989; 46(11 Suppl 2): 11-15.

Koppenhagen, FJ; Küpcü, Z; Wallner, G; Crommelin, DJ; Wagner, E; Storm, G; Kircheis, R. Sustained cytokine delivery for anticancer vaccination: liposomes as alternative for gene-transfected tumor cells. *Clin Cancer Res.* 1998; 4(8): 1881-1886.

Kuang, M; Peng, BG; Lu, MD. et al. Phase II randomized trial of autologous formalin-fixed tumor vaccine for postsurgical recurrence of hepatocellular carcinoma. *Clin Cancer Res* 2004; 10: 1574–1579.

Jiang, D; Premachandra, GS; Johnston, C; Hem, SL. Structure and adsorption properties of commercial calcium phosphate adjuvant. *Vaccine.* 2004; 23(5): 693-698.

Livingston, PO; Wong, GYC; Adluri, S; Tao, Y; Padavan, M; Parente, R; Hanlon, C; Helling, F; Ritter, G; Oettgen, HF; Old, LJ. Improved survival in AJCC stage III melanoma patients with GM2 antibodies: a randomized trial of adjuvant vaccination with GM2 ganglioside. *J. Clin. Oncol.* 1994; 12: 1036-1044.

Loibner, H; Eller, N; Groiss, F. et al. A randomized placebo-controlled phase II study with the cancer vaccine IGN101 in patients with epithelial solid organ tumors (IGN101/2–01). *Proc Am Soc Clin Oncol* 2004; 22: 14.

Lonchay, C; van der Bruggen, P; Connerotte, T; Hanagiri, T; Coulie, P; Colau, D; Lucas, S; Van Pel, A; Thielemans, K; van Baren, N; Boon T. Correlation between tumor regression and T cell responses in melanoma patients vaccinated with a MAGE antigen. *Proc Natl Acad Sci U S A.* 2004; 101(2): 14631-14638.

Maass, G; Schmidt, W; Berger, M; Schilcher, F; Koszik, F; Schneeberger, A; Stingl, G; Birnstiel, M.L; Schweighoffer, T. Priming of tumor-specific T-cells in the draining lymph nodes after immunization with interleukin-2 secreting tumor cells: Three consecutive stages may be required for successful tumor vaccination. *Proc. Natl. Acad. Sci. USA* 1995; 92: 5540-5544.

MacLean, GD; Reddish, MA; Koganty, RR. et al. Antibodies against mucin-associated sialyl-Tn epitopes correlate with survival of metastatic adenocarcinoma patients undergoing active specific immunotherapy with synthetic STn vaccine. *J Immunother Emphasis Tumor Immunol.* 1996; 19: 59–68.

MacLean, GD; Reddish, MA; Koganty, RR; Longenecker, BM. Antibodies against mucin-associated SialylTn epitopes correlate with survival of metastatic adenocarcinoma patients undergoing active specific immunotherapy with synthetic STn vaccine. *J. Immunother.* 1996; 19: 59-68.

Marchand, M; Punt, CJ; Aamdal, S; Escudier, B; Kruit, WH; Keilholz, U; Håkansson, L; van Baren, N; Humblet, Y; Mulders, P; Avril, MF; Eggermont, AM; Scheibenbogen, C; Uiters, J; Wanders, J; Delire, M; Boon, T. Stoter GImmunisation of metastatic cancer patients with MAGE-3 protein combined with adjuvant SBAS-2: a clinical report. *Eur J Cancer.* 2003; 39(1): 70-77.

Marincola, FM; Jaffee, EM; Hicklin, DJ; Ferrone, S. Escape of human tumors from T-cell recognition: molecular mechanisms and functional significance. *Adv. Immunol.* 2000; 74: 181-273.

Marotta, G; Frassoldati, A; Zinzani, P; Annino, L; Brugiatelli, M; Ambrosetti, A; Lenoci, M; Federico, M; Foa R, Lauria F; Italian Cooperative group for HCL (ICGHCL). Role of interferon-alpha administration after 2-deoxycoformycin in the treatment of hairy cell leukemia patients. *Eur J Haematol.* 2006; 77(2): 109-113.

Matzinger, P. The danger model: a renewed sense of self. *Science* 2002; 296: 301–305.

Mazzaferro, V; Coppa, J; Carrabba, MG. et al. Vaccination with autologous tumor-derived heat-shock protein gp96 after liver resection for metastatic colorectal cancer. *Clin Cancer Res.* 2003; 9: 3235–3245.

Mellstedt, H; Fagerberg, J; Frodin, JE. et al. Augmentation of the immune response with granulocyte-macrophage colony-stimulating factor and other hematopoietic growth factors. *Curr Opin Hematol .* 1999; 6: 169–175

Miles, D; Papazisis, K. Rationale for the clinical development of STn-KLH (Theratope) and anti-MUC-1 vaccines in breast cancer. *Clin Breast Cancer.* 2003; 3(4): 134-138.

Miles, DW; Towlson, KE; Graham, R; Reddish, M; Longenecker, BM; Taylor-Papadimitriou, J; Rubens, RD. A randomised phase II study of sialyl-Tn and DETOX-B adjuvant with or without cyclophosphamide pretreatment for the active specific immunotherapy of breast cancer. *Br J Cancer.* 1996; 74(8): 1292-1296.

Miller, JF; Morahan, G; nad Allison J. Cold Spring Harb. *Symp. Quant. Biol.* 1989; 2: 807-813.

Mosolits, S; Ullenhag, G; Mellstedt, H. Therapeutic vaccination in patients with gastrointestinal malignancies. A review of immunological and clinical results. *Ann Oncol.* 2005; 16(6): 847-862.

Naito, Y; Saito, K; Shiiba, K. et al. CD8+ T cells infiltrated within cancer cell nests as prognostic factor in human colorectal cancer. *Cancer res.* 1998; 58: 3491-3494.

Nakano, O; Sato, M; Naito, Y. et al. Proliferative activity of intratumoral CD8+ T-lymphocytes as a prognostic factor in human renal cell carcinoma: Clinicopathologic demonstration of antitumor immunity. *Cancer Res.* 2001; 61: 5132-5236.

Nauts, H; Fowler, G; Bogatko, F. A review of the influence of bacterial infection and of bacterial products (Coley's toxin) on malignant tumors in man; a critical analysis of 30 inoperable cases treated by Coley's mixed toxins, in which diagnosis was confirmed by microscopic examination selected for special study. *Acta Med. Scand.* 1953; 144: 1-103.

Nemunaitis, J; Jahan, T; Ross, H; Sterman, D; Richards, D; Fox, B; Jablons, D; Aimi, J; Lin, A. Hege K.Phase 1/2 trial of autologous tumor mixed with an allogeneic GVAX vaccine in advanced-stage non-small-cell lung cancer. *Cancer Gene Ther.* 2006; 13(6): 555-562.

Noguchi Y, Richards EC, Chen YT, Old LJ. Influence of interleukin 12 on p53 peptide vaccination against established Meth A sarcoma. *Proc Natl Acad Sci U S A.* 92(6):2219-23, 1995.)

Ochsenbein, AF; Sierro, S; Odermatt, B; Pericin, M; Karrer, U; Hermans, J; Hemmi, S; Hengartner, H; Zinkernagel, RM. Roles of tumor location, second signals and cross priming in cytotoxic T-cell induction. *Nature* 2001; 411: 1058-1064.

Ohashi, PS; Oehen, S; Buerki, K; Pircher, H; Ohashi, CT; Odermatt, B; Malissen, B; Zinkernagel, RM; Hengartner, H. Ablation of "tolerance" and induction of diabetes by virus infection in viral antigen transgenic mice. *Cell.* 1991; 65: 305-317.

Panelli, MC; White, R; Foster, M; Martin, B; Wang, E; Smith, K; Marincola, FM. Forecasting the cytokine storm following systemic interleukin (IL)-2 administration. *J. Translational Medicine.* 2004; 2: 17-31.

Pardoll, DM. Paracrine cytokine adjuvants in cancer immunotherapy. *Ann. Rev. Immunol.* 1995; 13: 399-415.

Parmiani, G; De Filippo, A; Pilla, L; Castelli, C; Rivoltini, L. Heat shock proteins gp96 as immunogens in cancer patients. *Int J Hyperthermia. 2006;* 22(3): 223-227.

Pham, HL; Ross, BP; McGeary, RP; Shaw, PN; Hewavitharana, AK; Davies, NM. Saponins from Quillaja saponaria Molina: isolation, characterization and ability to form immuno stimulatory complexes (ISCOMs). *Curr Drug Deliv.* 2006; 3(4): 389-397.

Plautz, G.E; Yang, Z.-Y; Wu, B.-Y; Gao, X; Huang, L; Nabel, G.J. Immunotherapy of malignancy by in vivo gene transfer into tumors. *Proc. Natl. Acad. Sci. USA.* 1993; 90: 4645-4649.

Porgador, A; Gansbacher, B; Bannerji, R. et al. Antimetastatic vaccination of tumor-bearing mice with IL-2 gene-inserted tumor cells. *Int. J. Cancer.* 1993; 53: 471-477.

Portielje, JE; Gratama, JW; van Ojik, HH; Stoter, G; Kruit, WH. IL-12: a promising adjuvant for cancer vaccination. *Cancer Immunol Immunother*. 2003; 52(3): 133-144.

Przepiorka, D; Srivastava, PK. Heat shock protein--peptide complexes as immunotherapy for human cancer. *Mol Med Today*. 1998; 4(11): 478-84.

Ragupathi, G; Cappello, S; Yi, SS; Canter, D; Spassova, M; Bornmann, WG; Danishefsky, SJ; Livingston, PO. Comparison of antibody titers after immunization with monovalent or tetravalent KLH conjugate vaccines. *Vaccine*. 2002; 20(7-8): 1030-1038.

Ragupathi, G; Koide, F; Livingston, PO; Cho, YS; Endo, A; Wan, Q; Spassova, MK; Keding, SJ; Allen, J; Ouerfelli, O; Wilson, RM; Danishefsky, SJ. Preparation and evaluation of unimolecular pentavalent and hexavalent antigenic constructs targeting prostate and breast cancer: a synthetic route to anticancer vaccine candidates. *J Am Chem Soc*. 2006; 128(8): 2715-2725.

Ramesh, M; Turner, LF; Yadav, R; Rajan, TV; Vella, AT; Kuhn, LT. Effects of the physico-chemical nature of two biomimetic crystals on the innate immune response. *Int Immunopharmacol*. 2007; 7(13): 1617-1629.

Rayman, P; Wesa, AK; Richmond, AL; Das, T; Biswas, K; Raval, G; Storkus, WJ; Tannenbaum, C; Novick, A; Bukowski, R; Finke, J. Effect of renal cell carcinomas on the development of type-1 T-cell responses. *Clin. Cancer Res*. 2004; 10: 6360-6366.

Reddish, MA; MacLean, GD; Poppema, S. et al. Pre-immunotherapy serum CA27.29 (MUC-1) mucin level and CD69+ lymphocytes correlate with effects of Theratope sialyl-Tn-KLH cancer vaccine in active specific immunotherapy. *Cancer Immunol Immunother*.1996; 42: 303–309.

Riethmuller, G; Schneider-Gadicke, E; Schlimok, G; Schmiegel, W; Raab, R; Hoffken, K; Gruber, R; Pichlmaier, H; Hirsche, H; Pichlmayr, R. et al. Randomized trial of monoclonal antibody for adjuvant therapy of resected Dukes' C colorectal carcinoma. German Cancer Aid 17-1A Study group. *Lancet*. 1994; 343: 1172-1174.

Rodolfo, M; Bassi, C; Salvi, C; Parmiani, G. Therapeutic use of a long-term cytotoxic T cell line recognizing a common tumor-associated antigen: the pattern of in vitro reactivity predicts the in vivo effect on different tumors. *Cancer Immunol. Immunother*. 1991; 34: 53-62.

Rosenberg, SA. Interleukin 2 for patients with renal cancer. *Nat Clin Pract Oncol*. 2007; 4(9): 497.

Rosenberg, SA; Yang, JC; Topalian, SL; Schwartzentruber, DJ; Weber, JS; Parkinson, DR; Seipp, CA; Einhorn, JH; White, DE. Treatment of 283 consecutive patients with metastatic melanoma or renal cell cancer using high-dose bolus interleukin. *JAMA*. 1994; 271(12): 907-913.

Rosenstein, M; Ettinghausen, SE; Rosenberg, SA. Extravasation of intravascular fluid mediated by the systemic administration of recombinant interleukin 2. *J Immunol*. 1986; 137(5): 1735-1742.

Sabbatini, PJ; Ragupathi, G; Hood, C; Aghajanian, CA; Juretzka, M; Iasonos, A; Hensley, ML; Spassova, MK; Ouerfelli, O; Spriggs, DR; Tew, WP; Konner, J; Clausen, H; Abu Rustum, N; Dansihefsky, SJ; Livingston, PO. Pilot study of a heptavalent vaccine-keyhole limpet hemocyanin conjugate plus QS-21 in patients with epithelial ovarian, fallopian tube, or peritoneal cancer. *Clin Cancer Res*. 2007; 13(14): 4170-4177.

Salgia, R; Lynch, T; Skarin, A; Lucca, J; Lynch, C; Jung, K; Hodi, FS; Jaklitsch, M; Mentzer, S; Swanson, S; Lukanich, J; Bueno, R; Wain, J; Mathisen, D; Wright, C; Fidias, P; Donahue, D; Clift, S; Hardy, S; Neuberg, D; Mulligan, R; Webb, I; Sugarbaker, D; Mihm, M; Dranoff, G. Vaccination with irradiated autologous tumor cells engineered to secrete granulocyte-macrophage colony-stimulating factor augments antitumor immunity in some patients with metastatic non-small-cell lung carcinoma. *J Clin Oncol.* 2003; 21(4): 624-630.

Samonigg, H; Wilders-Truschnig, M; Kuss, I. et al. A double-blind randomized-phase II trial comparing immunization with antiidiotype goat antibody vaccine SCV 106 versus unspecific goat antibodies in patients with metastatic colorectal cancer. *J Immunother.* 1999; 22: 481–488.

Sanchez, EQ; Marubashi, S; Jung, G; et al. De novo tumors after liver transplantation: A single institution experience. *Liver Transpl.* 2002; 8: 285-291.

Schellack, C; Prinz, K; Egyed, A; Fritz, JH; Wittmann, B; Ginzler, M; Swatosch, G; Zauner, W; Kast, C; Akira, S; von Gabain, A; Buschle, M; Lingnau, K. IC31, a novel adjuvant signaling via TLR9, induces potent cellular and humoral immune responses. *Vaccine.* 2006; 24(26): 5461-5472.

Schiller, JH; Pugh, M; Kirkwood, JM; Karp, D; Larson, M; Borden, E. Eastern cooperative group trial of interferon gamma in metastatic melanoma: an innovative study design. *Clin. Cancer Res.* 1996; 2: 29-36.

Schmidt, W; Schweighoffer, T; Herbst, E. et al. Cancer vaccines: The interleukin 2 dosage effect. *Proc. Natl. Acad. Sci. USA.* 1995; 92: 4711-4714.

Schumacher, K; Haensch, W; Roefzaad, C. et al. Prognostic significance of activated CD8+ T cell infiltrations within esophageal carcinomas. *Cancer Res.* 2001; 61: 3932-3936.

Seeber, SJ; White, JL; Hem, SL. Solubilization of aluminium-containing adjuvants by constituents of interstitial fluid. *J. Parenteral Sci. Technol.* 1991; 45: 1412-1416.

Settaf, A; Salzberg, M; Groiss, F; Eller, N; Schuster, M; Himmler, G; Kundi, M; Eckert, H; Loibner, H. A randomized placebo-controlled Phase II study with the cancer vaccine IGN101 in patients with epithelial cancers. *iSBTc 19th Annual Meeting, San Franscisco*, 4-7. 11. 2004

Singhal, A; Fohn, M; Hakomori, S-I. Induction of a α-N-acetylgalactosamine-O-serine/threonine (Tn) antigen-mediated cellular immune response for active immunotherapy in mice. *Cancer Res.* 1991; 51: 1406-1411.

Sjolander, A; Drane, D; Maraskovsky, E. Immune responses to ISCOM® formulations in animal and primate models. *Vaccine.* 2001; 19: 2661–2665.

Seubert, A; Monaci, E; Pizza, M; O'Hagan, DT; Wack, A. The adjuvants aluminum hydroxide and MF59 induce monocyte and granulocyte chemoattractants and enhance monocyte differentiation toward dendritic cells. *J Immunol.* 2008; 180(8): 5402-5412.

Slingluff, CL Jr; Yamshchikov, G; Neese, P; Galavotti, H; Eastham, S; Engelhard, VH; Kittlesen, D; Deacon, D; Hibbitts, S; Grosh, WW; Petroni, G; Cohen, R; Wiernasz, C; Patterson, JW; Conway, BP; Ross, WG. Phase I trial of a melanoma vaccine with gp100(280-288) peptide and tetanus helper peptide in adjuvant: immunologic and clinical outcomes. *Clin Cancer Res.* 2001; 7(10): 3012-3024.

Slovin, SF; Keding, SJ; Ragupathi, G. Carbohydrate vaccines as immunotherapy for cancer. *Immunol Cell Biol.* 2005; 83(4): 418-428.

Slovin, SF; Ragupathi, G; Fernandez, C; Diani, M; Jefferson, MP; Wilton, A; Kelly, WK; Morris, M; Solit, D; Clausen, H; Livingston, P; Scher, HI. A polyvalent vaccine for high-risk prostate patients: "are more antigens better?" *Cancer Immunol Immunother.* 2007; 56(12): 1921-1930.

Slovin, SF; Ragupathi, G; Fernandez, C; Jefferson, MP; Diani, M; Wilton, AS; Powell, S; Spassova, M; Reis, C; Clausen, H; Danishefsky, S; Livingston, P; Scher, HI. A bivalent conjugate vaccine in the treatment of biochemically relapsed prostate cancer: a study of glycosylated MUC-2-KLH and Globo H-KLH conjugate vaccines given with the new semi-synthetic saponin immunological adjuvant GPI-0100 OR QS-21. *Vaccine.* 2005; 23(24): 3114-3122.

Soiffer, R; Hodi, FS; Haluska, F; Jung, K; Gillessen, S; Singer, S; Tanabe, K; Duda, R; Mentzer, S; Jaklitsch, M; Bueno, R; Clift, S; Hardy, S; Neuberg, D; Mulligan, R; Webb, I; Mihm, M; Dranoff, G. Vaccination with irradiated, autologous melanoma cells engineered to secrete granulocyte-macrophage colony-stimulating factor by adenoviral-mediated gene transfer augments antitumor immunity in patients with metastatic melanoma. *J Clin Oncol.* 2003; 21(17): 3343-3350.

Sondak, VK; Sabel, MS; Mulé, JJ. Allogeneic and autologous melanoma vaccines: where have we been and where are we going? *Clin Cancer Res.* 2006; 12(7 Pt 2): 2337-2341.

Tamura, S. et al., Synergistic action of cholera toxin B subunit (and Escherichia coli heat-labile toxin B subunit) and a trace amount of cholera whole toxin as an adjuvant for nasal influenca vaccine. *Vaccine.* 1994; 12: 419-426.

Tamura, Y; Peng, P; Liu, K; Daou, M; Srivastava, PK. Immunotherapy of tumors with autologous tumor-derived heat shock protein preparations. *Science.* 1997; 278: 117-120.

Tartour, E; Benchetrit, F; Haicheur, N. et al. Synthetic and natural non-live vectors: rationale for their clinical development in cancer vaccine protocols. *Vaccine* 2002; 20(4): 32–39.

Tenderich, G; Deyerliong, W; Schulz, U. et al., Malignantneoplastic disorders following long-term immunosuppression after orthotopic heart transplantation. *Transplant. Proc.* 2001; 33: 3653-3655.

Thomas, M.C; Greten, T.F; Pardoll, D.M; Jaffee, E.M. Enhanced tumor protection by granulocyte-macrophage colony-stimulating factor expression at the site of an allogeneic vaccine. *Human Gene Ther.* 1998; 9: 835-843.

Travers, PJ; Arklie, JL; Trowsdale, J; Patillo, RA; Bodmer, WF. Lack of expression of HLA-ABC antigens in choriocarcinoma and other human tumor cell lines. *Natl. Cancer Inst. Monogr.* 1982; 60: 175-180.

Trinchieri, G. Function and clinical use of interleukin-12. *Curr Opin Hematol.* 1997; 4(1): 59-66.

Udono, H; Levey, DL; Srivastava, PK. Cellular requirements for tumor-specific immunity elicited by heat shock proteins: tumor rejection antigen gp96 primes CD8+ T cells in vivo. Proc Natl Acad Sci U S A. 1994; 91: 3077-3081.

Ulanova, M; Tarkowski, A; Hahn-Zoric, M; Hanson, LA. The common vaccine adjuvant aluminium hydroxide upregulates accessory properties of human monocytes via an interleukin-4-dependent mechanism. *Infect. Immun.* 2001; 69: 1151-1159.

Ullenhag, GJ; Frödin, JE; Mosolits, S; Kiaii, S; Hassan, M; Bonnet, MC; Moingeon, P; Mellstedt, H; Rabbani, H. Immunization of colorectal carcinoma patients with a recombinant canarypox virus expressing the tumor antigen Ep-CAM/KSA (ALVAC-KSA) and granulocyte macrophage colony- stimulating factor induced a tumor-specific cellular immune response. *Clin Cancer Res*. 2003; 9(7): 2447-2456.

Uyl-de Groot, CA; Vermorken, JB; Hanna, MG Jr; Verboom, P; Groot, MT; Bonsel, GJ; Meijer, CJ; Pinedo, HM. Immunotherapy with autologous tumor cell-BCG vaccine in patients with colon cancer: a prospective study of medical and economic benefits. *Vaccine*. 2005; 23(17-18): 2379-2387.

Van der Bruggen, P; Traversari, C; Chomez, P; Lurquin, C; DePlaen, E; Van den Eynde, B; Knuth, A; Boon, T. A gene encoding an antigen recognized by cytolytic T lymphocytes on a human melanoma. *Science* 1991; 254: 1643-1647.

Van Slooten, ML; Kircheis, R; Koppenhagen, FJ; Wagner, E; Storm, G. Liposomes as cytokine-supplement in tumor cell-based vaccines. *Int J Pharm*. 1999; 183(1): 33-36.

Vantomme, V; Dantinne, C; Amrani, N; Permanne, P; Gheysen, D; Bruck, C; Stoter, G; Britten, CM; Keilholz, U; Lamers, CH; Marchand, M; Delire, M; Guéguen, M. Immunologic analysis of a phase I/II study of vaccination with MAGE-3 protein combined with the AS02B adjuvant in patients with MAGE-3-positive tumors. *J Immunother*. 2004; 27(2): 124-135.

Vázquez-Lavista, LG; Flores-Balcázar, CH; Llorente, L. [The bacillus Calmette-Guérin as immunomodulator in bladder cancer][Article in Spanish] *Rev Invest Clin*. 2007; 59(2): 146-152.

Vermorken, JB; Claessen, AM; van Tinteren, H; et al. Active specific immunotherapy for stage II and stage III human colon cancer: a randomised trial. *Lancet*. 1999; 353: 345–350.

Waller, EK. The role of sargramostim (rhGM-CSF) as immunotherapy. *Oncologist*. 2007; 12(2): 22-26.

Wang, P; Kim, YJ; Navarro-Villalobos, M; Rohde, BD; Gin, DY. Synthesis of the potent immunostimulatory adjuvant QS-21A. *J Am Chem Soc*. 2005; 127(10): 3256-3257.

Watson, SA; Michaeli, D; Grimes, S; Morris, TM; Robinson, G; Varro, A; Justin, TA; Hardcastle, JD. Gastrimmune raises antibodies that neutralize amidated and glycine-extended gastrin-17 and inhibit the growth of colon cancer. *Cancer Res*. 1996; 56: 880-885.

Werdelin, O; Meldal, M; Jensen, T. Processing of glycans on glycoprotein and glycopeptide antigens in antigen-presenting cells. *Proc. Natl. Acad. Sci. USA*. 2002; 99: 9611-9613.

Werther, JL; Rivera-MacMurray, S; Bruckner, H; Tatematsu, M; Itzkowitz, SH. Mucin-associated sialosyl-Tn antigen expression in gastric cancer correlates with an adverse outcome. *Br. J. Cancer* 1994; 69: 613-616.

Yamamura, M; Modlin, RL; Ohmen, JD; and Moy, RL. Local expression of anti-inflammatory cytokines in cancer. J. Clin. Invest. 1993; 91: 1005-1010.

Yang, JC; Sherry, RM; Steinberg, SM; Topalian, SL; Schwartzentruber, DJ; Hwu, P; Seipp, CA; Rogers-Freezer, L; Morton, KE; White, DE; Liewehr, DJ; Merino, MJ; Rosenberg, SA. Randomized study of high-dose and low-dose interleukin-2 in patients with metastatic renal cancer. *J Clin Oncol*. 2003; 21(16): 3127-3132.

Zatloukal, K; Schneeberger, A; Berger, M. et al. Elicitation of a systemic and protective antimelanoma immune response by an IL-2 based vaccine. *J. Immunol.* 1995; 154: 3406-3419.

Zhang, H; Zhang, S; Cheung, NK; Ragupathi, G; Livingston, PO. Antibodies can eradicate cancer micrometastases. Cancer Res. 1998; 58: 2844-2849.

Zhang, L; Conejo-Garcia, JR; Katsaros, D. et al. Intratumoral T cells, recurrence, and survival in epithelial ovarian cancer. *N. Engl. J. Med.* 2003; 348: 203-213.

Zhang, S; Zhang, SH; Cordon-Cardo, C; Reuter, VE; Singgal, AK; Lloyd, KO; Livingston, PO. Selection of tumor antigens as targets for immune attack using immunohistochemistry. II. Blood group-related antigens. *Int. J. Cancer.* 1997; 73: 50-56.

Zhang, S; Walberg, LA; Ogata, S; Itzkowitz, SH; Koganty, RR; Reddish, M; Gandhi, SS; Longenecker, BM; Lloyd, KO; Livingston, PO. Immune sera and monoclonal antibodies define two configurations for the sialylTn tumor antigen. *Cancer Res.* 1995; 55: 3364-3368.

Zurbriggen, R; Glück, R. Immunogenicity of IRIV-versus alum-adjuvanted diphtheria and tetanus toxoid vaccines in influenza primed mice. *Vaccine* 1999; 17: 1301–1305.

In: Immunologic Adjuvant Research
Editor: Antonio H. Benvenuto

ISBN 978-1-60692-399-3
© 2009 Nova Science Publishers, Inc.

Chapter 2

TLR Agonists as Immune Adjuvants

Yanal Murad and Bara Sarraj
1. Department of Experimental Surgery, Duke University, Durham, NC.
2. Department of Lab Medicine, Children's Hospital Boston, Boston, MA.

Abstract

The immune system can be broadly divided into innate and adaptive, bridged by antigen-presenting cells, like dendritic cells. While the adaptive immunity is specific and requires antigen presentation, the innate immune system recognizes foreign pathogens in a non-specific manner, and then responds through effectors like cytokines. Toll like receptors (TLRs) are part of the innate immune system, and they belong to the pattern recognition receptors (PRR) family, which is designed to recognize and bind certain molecules that are restricted to pathogens, like LPS and CpG. Different TLR signals converge through few common adapter proteins to relay their signals, a process that results in the activation of several genes essential for mounting an immune response. The wide distribution of TLRs on hematopoietic and non-hematopoietic cells, and their high potential for activating the host immune system makes TLR ligands great adjuvant candidates. They will elicit their function on a wide variety of cells, and stimulate both the innate and adaptive immune systems. Thus, TLRs are considered as major targets for the development of agonists that could serve as adjuvants and agents of immunotherapy. Several of these TLR agonists, including TLR2, TLR4, TLR7 and TLR9 agonists are being developed and tested in clinical trials. This chapter reviews the development of these agonists for clinical use, and potential future applications.

Introduction

Adjuvants are immune response or drug action enhancers that, along with antigens, comprise the primary components of effective vaccines. Major components of adjuvants are bacterial or viral extracts, mineral oils and aluminum hydroxide metal [1]. Adjuvants mostly prime antigen-presenting myeloid dendritic cells (mDCs) and interferon-producing plasmacytoid DCs (pDCs). Known examples of adjuvants are Freund's and Bacille Calmette-Guérin (BCG) [1]. The immune system is divided into innate and adaptive, connected by antigen-presenting cells. The adaptive immunity, which is highly sophisticated, and present only in higher organisms, detects non-self antigens and pathogens through recognition of peptide antigens using antigen receptors expressed on the surface of B and T cells. In contrast, the innate immune system is conserved among multicellular organisms, and is designed to recognize pathogen-associated molecular patterns (PAMPs), which are restricted to pathogens and absent in vertebrates, through pattern recognition receptors (PRR).

PRRs are germ line encoded molecules, present on different immune cells and are divided into intracellular and extracellular innate receptors [2, 3]. Characterized intracellular innate receptors (TLR-independent) include anti-bacterial nucleotide-domain oligomerization (NOD)-like receptors (NLR) and anti-viral retinoic-acid-inducible gene I (RIG)-like receptors (RLR) [4-6]. Among the best known and studied PRRs are Toll Like Receptors (TLRs). TLRs were first discovered in vertebrates on the basis of their homology with Drosophila Toll protein, a molecule that stimulates the production of antimicrobial proteins in *Drosophila melanogaster* [7, 8]. TLRs belong to the Toll superfamily, which also include the IL-1 receptor (IL-1R) and IL-18R. There are at least 12 members of the TLR family in vertebrates discovered to date (9 in humans) (Table 1).

Table 1. TLRs, agonists and adjuvants

TLR	Ligands	Expression/location	Adjuvant
TLR1	Lipoproteins	Cell surface	Pam3Cys*
TLR2	Lipoteichoic acid	intracellular Cell surface	Pam3Cys/MALP2/OspA*
TLR3	dsRNA	intracellular	PolyI:C
TLR4	LPS	intracellular Cell surface	MPL
TLR5	Flagellin	intracellular Cell surface	Flagellin
TLR6	Lipoproteins	Cell surface	MALP-2*
TLR7	Viral ssRNA	intracellular	Imidazoquinolins/polyU**
TLR8	Viral ssRNA	intracellular	Imidazoquinolins/polyU**
TLR9	CpG DNA	intracellular	CpG ODNs (table 3)

* TLR2 in dimerization with TLR1/TLR6/unknown, respectively.
** TLR7/8 heterodimer.
Monophosphoryl lipid A, MPL; *Mycoplasma* macrophage-activating lipopeptide 2, MALP-2; Outer surface lipoprotein, OspA;

Table 2. TLR cell distribution [1, 2, 9]

TLR	Cells
TLR1	Leukocytes
TLR2	Gr, Mf, NK, DC, T, B, Fb, Ep.
TLR3	Human and murine mDCs
TLR4	Gr, Mf, NK, DC, T, B, Fb, Ep.
TLR5	Ep, DCs
TLR6	DCs
TLR7	Immune cells, human pDCs, murine pDCs
TLR8	Human monocytes and myeloid DCs
TLR9	Immune cells, human pDCs and B cells, murine mDCs and pDCs

The wide distribution of TLRs (from DCs, macrophages, and NK cells to B and T cells and even endothelial and epithelial cells), and their high potential for activating the host immune system makes the TLR ligands great adjuvant candidates, since they will elicit their function on a wide variety of cells, and stimulate both the innate and adaptive immune system (Table 2). In fact, TLRs and other PRRs are widely distributed on haematopoietic and non-haematopoietic cells, with each cell type expressing a typical pattern of PRRs. This pattern of expression is further modulated or modified by the activation, maturation or differentiation of the cells [3].

Granulocyte, Gr; macrophage, Mf; natural killer cell, NK; dendritic cell, DC; fibroblast, Fb; epithelial cell, Ep; myeloid DC, mDC; plasmacytoid DC, pDC.

Structure

TLRs are single-pass transmembrane proteins with an N-terminal Leucine-rich repeats (LRRs), a transmembrane domain, and a C-terminal cytoplasmic domain.

The extracellular domain of TLRs, which can recognize specific pathogen components, contains 19–25 tandem copies of the LRR motif, each of which is 24–29 amino acids in length [10], but despite the conservation among LRR domains, different TLRs can recognize several structurally unrelated ligands [11-13]. TLR structures show high similarity to that of the interleukin-1 receptor (IL-1R) family, and share IL-1R intracellular domain, a conserved region of ~200 amino acids in their cytoplasmic tails, which is known as the Toll/IL-1R (TIR) domain [14, 15].

The history of adjuvants that target TLRs date back to William Coley, who used bacterial extracts for the treatment of cancer [16]. More recently, many established and experimental vaccines incorporate TLR ligands in prophylactic vaccines against infectious diseases, as well as in therapeutic immunization for diseases like cancer. The engagement of TLR signaling pathways maybe used to trigger an adaptive immune response that could boost vaccine responses [9]. It has been reported that in most cases, signaling through TLRs will favor a Th1-type immune response, which is needed for the protection against most pathogens [17]

Signaling:

TLR Activation

The activation of TLRs begins with the ligand binding to extracellular LRRs and, either through receptor oligomerization and/or induction of a conformational change across the plasma membrane; this will induce the recruitment/activation of adapter proteins through the Toll/IL-1 Receptor (TIR) domain.

TLRs recruit a specific combination of TIR-domain-containing adaptors, including myeloid differentiation primary response gene 88 (MyD88), TIR-containing adaptor protein/MyD88-adaptor-like (TIRAP/MAL), TIR-domain-containing adaptor inducing interferon-β (IFN-β)/TIR-domain-containing adaptor molecule 1 (TRIF/TICAM1) and TRIF-related adaptor molecule 2/TIR-domain-containing adaptor molecule (TRAM/TICAM2) [14, 18, 19] (Figure 1).

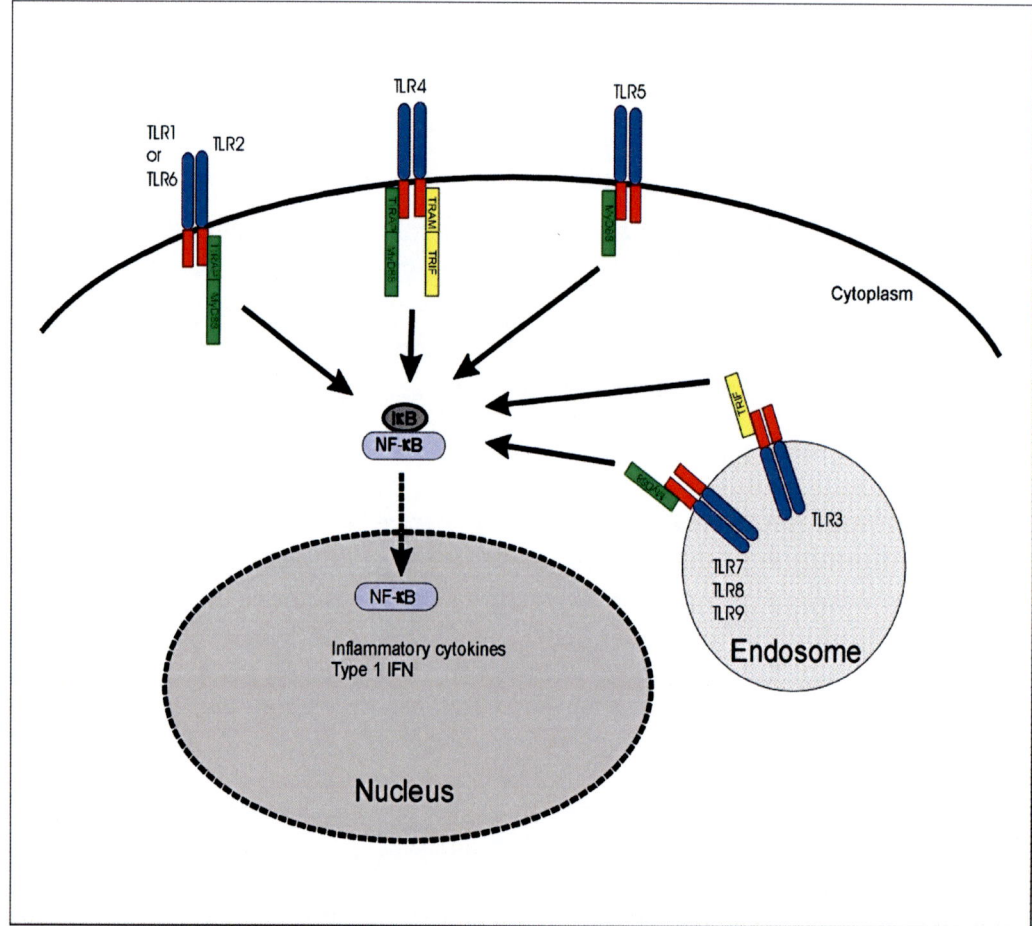

Figure 1. Overview of different TLR signaling pathways, which leads to the activation of NF-κB, through either MyD88 or TRIF mediated pathways. All TLRs signal through MyD88, except for TLR3 and TLR 2 subfamily (TLR 1, TLR2 and TLR6), which signal through TRIF. TLR4 can signal through either pathway. Different TLR ligands are summarized in table 1.

All TLR molecules use MyD88 for signaling, except TLR3, which uses TRIF instead [20]. MyD88 serves as the sole signal relay in TLR5, TLR7, and TLR9. That was indicated when it was shown that NF-κB activation and inflammatory cytokine induction is defective in MyD88-deficient mice [21, 22]. However, the response is normal in mice deficient for TIRAP, TRIF or TRAM, indicating that MyD88 is used as the sole adaptor by these TLRs. TLR2 requires TIRAP as an adaptor to bridge between MyD88 and TLR2 [23, 24], while TLR4 uses all of these adaptors (MyD88, TRIF, TRAM, and TIRAP) for signaling [23, 25, 26]. These adapters lead to the activation of canonical IKKβ-dependent complexes, degradation of IκBα and IκBβ, and liberation of, primarily, RelA and c-Rel nuclear factor-κB (NF-κB) components (Figure 1).

Myd88-Dependent Pathway

The MyD88-dependent pathway signals via MyD88, IRAK, and TRAF6 and leads to NF-κB activation. MyD88 is composed of two domains: a TIR domain and a death domain. Upon TLR activation, through its death domain, MyD88 interacts with the death domains of members of the IRAK (IL-1 receptor-associated kinase) family of protein kinases, including IRAK1, IRAK2, IRAK4 and IRAK-M [14, 18]. It is believed that all MyD88- utilizing TLRs directly recruit MyD88, except for TLR2 and TLR4, which use a TIR domain containing adaptor (TIRAP) to bridge MyD88 to TLR. Once phosphorylated, IRAKs dissociate from MyD88 and interact with TRAF6, a member of the TRAF family. TRAF6, an E3 ligase, forms a complex with Ubc13 and Uev1A to promote the synthesis of lysine 63-linked polyubiquitin chains, which in turn activate TAK1, a MAPKKK [27]. This activation of TAK1 will lead to the activation of IKK complex, and eventually NF-κB, through yet undefined mediators [28, 29].

Myd88-Independent (TRIF-Dependent) Pathway

This pathway, also called TRIF-dependent pathway, activates NF-κB through the RIP1/TRAF6–TAK1–IKKα/β pathway. This pathway was discovered when MyD88$^{-/-}$ cells displayed partial NF-κB activation when exposed to LPS [30]. Also, when cells are stimulated through TLR3 and TLR4, TRIF will mediate the activation of NF-κB in the absence of MyD88 [31]. For TLR3, all downstream signaling appears to be TRIF-mediated, while TLR4 can signal through either MyD88 or TRIF pathways.

NF-κB Activation

All TLR family receptors trigger their effects through the activation of NF-κB dependent and interferon (IFN)-regulatory factor (IRF)-dependent signaling pathways through the MyD88- or TRIF-dependent pathway, or both [32]. NF-κB molecule functions are enormously diverse leading to activation of a wide variety of genes. Normally, NF-κB activates anti-apoptotic genes, where it plays a prosurvival as well as proinflammatory roles. One of the primary roles of NF-κB is the control of the transcription of cytokines, antimicrobial effectors, and genes that regulate the various aspects of the innate and adaptive immune system [33, 34].

NF-κB family in mammals is composed of 5 members: RelA (p65), RelB, cytoplasmic (C)-Rel, p105 (NF-κB1), and p100 (NF-κB2). The different members of the NF- κB family form dimeric transcription factors (homo or hetero), using their Rel-Homology domain (RHD), which is a highly conserved DNA-binding/dimerization domain [35], and bind to DNA sequences known as κB sites (5'-GGGRNNYYCC-3'; R, purine; Y, pyrimidine; N, any nucleotide) to regulate the expression of genes involved in many processes, including innate and adaptive immunity, inflammation, and cancer progression [35]. NF-κB dimers are usually sequestered in the cytoplasm in an inactive form by molecules of the inhibitor of NF-κB (IκB) family, which through direct interaction with NF-κB, masks the nuclear localization signal. The IκB family consists of seven members, IκBα, IκBβ, IκB γ, IκB ε, IκB ζ, Bcl-3, and IκBNS. While IκBα, IκB β, IκB γ, IκB ε bind NF-κB protein in the cytoplasm, IκB ζ, Bcl-3, and IκBNS are nuclear proteins that regulate the activity of NF-κB.

The stimulation of TLRs triggers the canonical activation pathway through the phosphorylation of specific serine residues of IκB proteins by a multiprotein IKK complex, which consists of two catalytic components, IKKα and IKKβ, and a regulatory component, NEMO (NF-κB essential modifier, aka IKK γ). Phosphorylated IκB proteins are subsequently polyubiquitinated and degraded by the 26S proteasome, allowing NF-κB to move into the nucleus. The most frequently activated form of NF-κB in TLR signaling is a heterodimer of RelA and p50.

The non-canonical (or alternative) pathway of NF-κB activation is largely for activation of p100/RelB complexes during B-and T-cell organ development. This pathway differs from the canonical pathway in that only certain receptor signals (e.g., Lymphotoxin B (LTβ), B-cell activating factor (BAFF), CD40) activate this pathway, and it proceeds through an IKK complex that contains two IKKα subunits (but not NEMO) [35]. The receptor binding in the non canonical pathway leads to activation of NIK, the NF-κB-inducing kinase, which phosphorylates and activates an IKKα complex that in turn phosphorylates two serine residues adjacent to the ankyrin repeat C-terminal IκB domain of p100, leading to its partial proteolysis and liberation of the p52/RelB complex. Both p105 and p100 contain C-terminal ankyrin repeats, which function as IκB -like proteins, binding to their own RHD to prevent nuclear translocation. Ubiquitin-dependent proteolytic degradation of the C-terminal region of p105 and p100 results in the generation of mature p50 and p52 [36].

TLRS and Neutrophils

Neutrophils are the first to arrive at the site of infection where they secrete cytokines/chemokines, reactive oxygen species, and proteases and phagocytose pathogens, thus representing an essential pillar of innate immunity that TLR initial function belongs to. As neutrophils are predominant in numerous pathologic conditions such as pneumonia, rheumatoid arthritis and ischemia/reperfusion, exploring the role of TLRs, especially TLR4, in neutrophil pathology is expanding. Tsuda et al. divided neutrophils into three groups in terms of cell susceptibility to methicilin-resistant staphylococcus aureus or MRSA; all these distinctly characterized groups expressed TLR2/4 [37]. Human neutrophils express all TLRs but TLR3 [38]. Neutrophils express low levels of TLR2/4 and CD14 and its response to LPS (L-selectin shedding, Mac-1 upregulation and cell survival) is monocyte-dependent [39]. Delayed apoptosis of neutrophils might be TLR/CD14-induced and caspase 3-mediated [40]. Another study showed that TLR2,4,7,8 and 9 ligation was comparably effective in delaying apoptosis of human PMNs in vitro [41]. TLR4 was involved in oxidative burst promotion by murine neutrophils [42] and in enhanced chemokine-induced neutrophil migration by modulating the chemokine receptor expression [43]. Neutrophil TLR2/4 activation lead to changes in adhesion molecule expression, IL-8 and respiratory burst, and CXCR1/2 decrease [44, 45]. TLR agonists primed neutrophils to produce cytokines and superoxide radicals, shed L-selectin, enhance phagocytosis but impair chemotaxis to IL-8 [46]. LPS instillation in the lungs of BALB/c mice induced GM-CSF-augmented TNF, MIP-2 and TNF production and neutrophilia [47]. However, mice susceptibility to Pseudomonas pneumonia was MyD88-dependent, but TLR2/4-independent [48, 49]. In addition, neutrophil infiltrates were reduced in TLR4 KO mouse liver post ischemia/reperfusion [50].

TLRS and Phosphoinositide-3-Kinase (Pi3k)

PI3K is an enzyme that produces phosphotidylinositol (3,4,5) trisphosphate (PIP3), a second messenger that leads to activation of downstream effector enzymes resulting in cell growth, survival, proliferation and motility. Therefore, it is essential to consider the interaction between these two major pathways (TLR and PI3K) and the resultant effects on the cell. PI3K activation has been observed after TLR ligation and, in general, negatively regulates TLR-mediated proinflammatory effects [51]. PI3K suppressed IL-12 Th1 response early at TLR activation [52], but augmented human pDC IFN-β production [53] and viral resistance by murine macrophages [54]. In addition, PI3K was found to suppress TLR3/4-induced, TRIF-dependent IFN-β production [55]. Whereas PI3K suppressed TLR5-mediated proinflammatory processes in vitro as well as in vivo [56], its blockade in human colonic epithelial cells reduced TLR5-mediated interleukin-8 production [57]. Wortmannin, a PI3K inhibitor, enhanced TLR-dependent expression of induced nitric oxide synthase (iNOS) in a cell line of mouse macrophages [58]; further, PTEN, a PI3K negative regulator, enhanced murine macrophage capability to clear intracellular Leishmania parasites [59]. TLR-dependent protective effects after murine hearts underwent ischemia/reperfusion were found mediated by PI3K [60]. TLR agonists were shown to delay apoptosis of human blood PMNs in a PI3K-dependent manner [41]. Staphylococcus aureus stimulated TLR2 in human THP1 and 293 cells and lead to NFκB activation in an IκBα-independent manner through the recruitment of active Rac-1 and PI3K to TLR2 cytosolic domain [61].

TLRs Agonists as Adjuvants

Prevention of infectious diseases through immunization was discovered and mentioned in the late 18th century, and is considered as one of the greatest achievements of modern medicine. Nonetheless, scientists are still facing considerable challenges for improving the efficacy of vaccines, whether it is for the development of new prophylactic vaccines for infectious agents, or for therapeutic immunization for noninfectious diseases such as cancer [9]. Regardless of the vaccine target, successful immunization results in activation of adaptive immunity, which might be accomplished, in part, through stimulation of the TLRs. The involvement of TLR pathways in activating adaptive immunity and vaccine responses is well established, and is explained by the control exerted by TLRs over the activation of adaptive immunity [62]. This control is mediated through several mechanisms, including TLR-mediated activation of dendritic cells (DCs) by upregulating chemokine, MHC and costimulatory receptors, producing cytokines and chemokines, suppression of T regulatory cells (T_{regs}) and reversal of tolerance [1, 9].

Cross-Priming of Cd8 T Cells

DCs can display exogenously internalized antigens on MHC class I molecules to CD8 T cells, a process termed cross-priming. Cross priming is very important in terms of vaccination against intracellular antigens that CD8 T cells will efficiently eliminate [9]. Murine DCs had been shown to cross present dsRNA or CpG to CTLs in vivo [63, 64].

How do TLRS Agonists Stimulate Adaptive Immunity?

We summarize here some of the mechanisms TLR agonists are thought to work to stimulate adaptive immunity

- IL-12 and Th1 responses

The stimulation of TLRs, in most instances, will favor the development a Th1 type of response, which is required for the protection against most pathogens [9, 65]. Also, it seems that IL-12 plays an important role in this process and in the stimulation of adaptive immunity [17, 66]. The synergistic effects of certain TLR ligands are marked by the production of IL-12 p70 (the active form of IL12), while stimulation of DCs with a single TLR ligand will normally induce negligible levels of biologically active IL12 [3, 67].

- Reversal of tolerance

Several studies have shown that the engagement of TLRs can overcome peripheral tolerance leading to specific CTL responses in therapeutic tumor vaccines, thus enhancing the vaccine efficiency [68-70]. Tolerance through T_{regs} (CD^+ $CD25^+$) can be overcome by stimulating TLRs on DCs, which was found to be dependent on IL-6 production, since $IL6^{-/-}$ mice were not able to prime pathogen-specific T cells in the presence of T_{reg} cells [9, 68].

Moreover, Stimulation of TLR8 on T_{reg} cells was found to reverse their suppression function [70].

- Upregulation of co-stimulatory molecules

Activation of TLRs leads to the upregualtion of several costimulatory molecules, like CD40, CD80, CD86, and CD70, on antigen presenting cells [62], which has been shown to improve vaccine efficacy [71-73]. Moreover, TLR activation will lead to DC maturation, and accumulation of MHC class II and antigen complexes on the cell surface [74, 75].

TLR Agonists in Clinical Use

TLR2

TLR2 recognizes a variety of microbial components, including lipoproteins from pathogens including Gram-negative bacteria, Mycoplasma and spirochets [76-78], peptidoglycan and lipoteichoic acid from Gram-positive bacteria [79-82], Lipoarabinomannan from mycobacteria [81-83] and several other microbial components from other microorganisms [84]. Probably the best known TLR2 agonist is the outer-surface lipoprotein (OspA) of *Borrelia burgdorferi*, which has been used as a vaccine for Lyme disease [85]. It has been hypothesized that OspA signals through TLR1/TLR2 heterodimer, since neither $TLR1^{-/-}$ nor $TLR2^{-/-}$ mice were able to mount a protective immune response after OspA vaccination; also, low responders to the vaccine were shown to have low surface expression of TLR1, but unchanged expression of TLR2 [86].

Another aspect of TLR2 ligand recognition involves interaction with other TLRs, including TLR1 and TLR6. Several reports suggested cooperation between TLR2 and TLR6, including co-immunoprecipitation of the two proteins [87], or the recognition of macrophage activating lipopeptide (MALP-2) only in the presence of both TLR2 and TLR6 [87]. MALP-2 is a synthetic lipopeptide with two long chain fatty acid ester residues that signals through TLR2 (associated with TLR6), activates nuclear transcription factor NF-κB, induces the synthesis of a number of cytokines and chemokines, depending on its target cell, and induces maturation of dendritic cells [88].

TLR4

One of the best studied interactions between a microbial pathogen-associated molecular pattern and a TLR is the recognition of lipopolysaccharide (LPS), the major component of the outer membrane of Gram-negative bacteria, by TLR4. It is known that the adjuvant activity of bacterial cell walls is responsible for their ability to activate the innate immune system through a cognate receptor. LPS, the TLR4 ligand, has been experimentally shown to be a potent adjuvant for vaccines, although its extreme toxicity prevents its use in humans. The adjuvant effect of LPS is solely dependent on TLR4-mediated, MyD88-dependent signaling. The dependence of LPS signaling on a single protein was revealed by the identification, in 1965, of a remarkable phenotype in mice marked by a very specific and profound insensitivity to LPS. The phenotype was first observed in mice of the C3H/HeJ strain, and neither the lethal effect of LPS nor any of the cellular effects of LPS occurred in these mice. This included the well-known adjuvant effect of LPS [89].

LPS is one of the most potent inducers of the immune system, and it was revealed later how it is recognized by a complex cascade of extracellular "pattern recognition receptors", which chaperone the LPS from the bacterial membrane to the transmembrane receptor TLR4. Two additional proteins have been identified that interact with TLR4 and are implicated in LPS recognition, MD-2 and CD14. MD-2 is a secreted molecule that physically interacts with TLR4. CD14 is a glycosylphosphatidylinositol-linked membrane protein (devoid of a cytoplasmic signaling domain) with LPS binding activity. Collectively TLR4, MD-2, and CD14 form a trimolecular LPS receptor complex [90, 91]. It is interesting to notice that TLR4 is the only known TLR which can utilize all five TIR- domain-containing adaptor proteins: MyD88, TIRAP, TRIF, TRAM, and SARM [19].

The lipid A portion of LPS was shown to be responsible for both the adjuvant and the toxic properties of LPS [92, 93]. Monophosphoryl lipid A (MPL) was developed by Ribi and co-workers as an attenuated derivative of LPS that lacks many of the endotoxic properties of the parent molecule and yet retains potent adjuvant and immunostimulating activities [94]. It was found that the removal of the phosphate group from the reducing end sugar of the lipid A disaccharide decreased the toxicity of the molecule 100 to 1000 folds without affecting the immunostimulating activity. The resulting derivative, which had only one phosphate group, was called monophosphoryl lipid A [94-96].

Subsequently, it was determined that removal of an ester-linked fatty acid group from the 3-position further reduced the pyrogenic properties without substantially affecting the adjuvant properties. The resulting 3-*O*-deacylated monophosphoryl lipid A (MPL), which is isolated and structurally derivatized from LPS of *Salmonella minnesota* R595, has proven to be a safe and effective vaccine adjuvant [97, 98]. In 1981, Takayama *et al.* isolated a nontoxic lipid A fraction, inducing tumor and metastases regression in animal models: ONO-4007 (sodium 2-deoxy-2-[3S-(9-phenylnonanoyloxy) tetradecanoyl] amino-3-O-(9-phenylnonanoyl)-Dglucopyranose 4-sulphate), developed by Ono Pharmaceutical Co (Osaka, Japan) [99]. Several animal studies also showed that ONO-4007 had remarkable and selective efficacy against TNF-α-sensitive tumors [100, 101]. Other partial agonists for TLR4, like DT-5461, SDZ MLR 953 and GLA-60, have been described, and although their development as anticancer agents was discontinued, their pharmacological profile deserves to be considered [102-104].

TLR5

TLR5 recognizes the bacterial protein flagellin, a 55-kDa monomeric protein constituent of flagella, which is the motility apparatus used by many microbial pathogens. The major protein constituent of bacteria flagella is also a potent activator of the innate immune responses [105]. The purification of culture supernatants of *Listeria monocytogenes* containing TLR5-stimulating activity led to the identification flagellin as the active component [105]. TLR5 is expressed by epithelial cells, monocytes, and immature DCs.

Biochemical analysis of *Salmonella* flagellin revealed that both conserved domains within both N- and C-termini of the protein are important in inducing proinflammatory responses in cultured intestinal epithelial cells [106, 107]. Recent studies also suggested that the hypervariable domain is not involved in proinflammatory activation. A recombinantly expressed flagellin mutant, in which the central hypervariable domain was deleted, was shown not to detract from its ability to induce NF-κB signaling, suggesting that the highly conserved N and C termini are sufficient for TLR5 activation [107]. A more recent study mapped the precise sequences responsible for the activity of flagellin on both the C- and N-termini of the protein [108].

CBLB502, a TLR5 agonist peptide, was found to protect against both major acute radiation toxicities of the hematopoietic system (HP) and gastrointestinal tract (GI). It was also found to reduce radiation toxicity without diminishing the therapeutic antitumor effect of radiation and without promoting radiation-induced carcinogenicity [109]. The results from this paper suggest that TLR5 agonists may be valuable as both adjuvants for cancer radiotherapy and protectants or mitigators for radiation emergencies [109]. In another study, a recombinant protein vaccine that was developed for West Nile virus, elicited a strong WNV-E-specific immunoglobulin G antibody response that neutralized viral infectivity and conferred protection against a lethal WNV challenge in C3H/HeN mice. The vaccine was designed by fusing a modified version of bacterial flagellin (STF2 Delta) to the EIII domain of the WNV envelope protein [110-112].

TLR7/8

TLR 7 and 8 were originally found to be expressed intracellularly and both interact with imidazoquinoline as a ligand in vitro. It has been suggested that TLR 7 and 8 differ in cell targets and cytokine production [113], but both induce the immune response to ssRNA human parechovirus 1 [114] and group B coxsackieviruses [115]. Both receptors are expressed on human bone marrow progenitor cells and ligation results in myeloid lineage differentiation [116]. TLR7 is also expressed on the surface of chronic lymphocytic leukemia cells [117]. Imiquimod, a synthetic TLR7 (porcine TLR7/8 [118]) agonist, is being used topically to treat a number of human pathological conditions such as genital warts and basal cell carcinoma. Imiquimod enhanced anti-melanoma vaccine effects in mice [119] and probably empowered DCs effector functions in basal cell carcinoma patients [120]. Further, a cryosurgery/imiquimod combined treatment of murine tumor had better curative outcome than cryosurgery alone [121]. Isatoribine, a selective TLR7 agonist, reduced plasma hepatitis C viral load in humans [122]. TLR7 had been suggested to be involved in murine autoimmunity and DC dysregulation [123, 124]. 852A, a specific TLR 7 agonist, is in phase I and II trial for advanced cancer patients [125, 126]. Treatment with S-28463, an imiquimod family member reduced allergic asthma in mice and associated symptoms in rats [127, 128] and TLR7/8 dual agonist 3M-011 protected rats against H3N2 influenza virus [129].

TLR9

Among the different TLRs, probably the greatest interest now revolves around TLR9, which recognizes bacterial and viral DNA with unmethylated CpG motifs in double stranded DNA (CpG DNA). TLR9 (in common with other members of the TLR family, including TLR3 and TLR7) is localized to the endosomal and lysosomal compartments within the cells, and is expressed primarily in B cells and pDCs [130-132].

The activation of TLR9 on pDCs induces the secretion of IFN-α, which drives the migration of pDCs to the marginal zone of lymph nodes, where they stimulate T cells [133]. Stimulation of TLR9 on human B cells induces proliferation, enhanced antigen specific antibody production, and IFN-α production. TLR9 activation, along with B cell antigen receptor, induces naïve B cell differentiation into plasma cells. Activation of TLR9 alone will drive the differentiation of memory B cells into plasma cells [134].

Three classes of CpG oligonucleotide ligands for TLR9 have been described, and can be distinguished by different sequence motifs and different abilities to stimulate IFN- α secretion and maturation of pDCs [135]. These structurally distinct classes of CpG ODN are class A, B and C. Class A, also known as type D, has a backbone made of phosphodiester bonds. This class has poly-G motifs flanking a central palindromic

sequence. This class strongly induces IFN-α secretion from pDCs, induces pDC maturation, but is a weak stimulator of B cell proliferation [136, 137]. Class B CpG ODN, also known as type K, includes the most studied TLR9 agonist, CpG-7909. This class has a phosphorothioate backbone and is a weak inducer of IFN-α secretion but a strong stimulator of B cell proliferation and pDC maturation. The third class, known as class C, has intermediate immune properties between classes A and B, where it induces both IFN-α secretion and B cell stimulation. This class also has a phosphorothioate backbone, and its sequence combines structural elements of both CpG ODN-A and CpG ODN-B. The most potent sequence M362, contains a 5′ end 'TCGTCG' motif and a 'GTCGTT' motif; both are present in CpG ODN-B (CPG-7909) and a palindromic sequence characteristic for CpG ODN-A (ODN 2216) [138, 139].

Short synthetic ODNs containing the immune stimulatory CpG motifs (CpG ODNs) have been used as a vaccine adjuvant in the treatment of cancer, asthma, allergies and infections [135, 140]. Several companies, such as Pfizer, Coley, Dynavax, and Idera, have produced CpG ODNs for clinical use (Table 3). A number of CpG ODNs have been or are being currently tested in multiple phase II and III trials as adjuvants to cancer vaccines and in combination with other conventional cancer therapies [140, 141]

TLR9 agonist CpG ODN treatment shifts the Th1/Th2 cytokine balance towards dominance of Th1 cytokines with increased synthesis of IgG2a, IFN, IL-6 and IL-12. This shift in cytokine balance makes CpG ODN useful for use in the treatment of several conditions where this balance is skewed towards a Th2 type reaction, in addition to its use as an adjuvant in vaccination protocols. Overproduction of Th2 cytokines and overexpression of IgE is the hallmark of allergic reactions[142], so the Th1-biased immune effect of CpG ODN has been applied in the development of allergy vaccines. A conjugate of CpG ODN to ragweed allergen has been evaluated as an allergy vaccine in allergic patients [143]. The immune response was successfully redirected towards a nonallergic and noninflammatory Th1 type, with a significant clinical benefit and reduced allergic symptoms.

CpG ODN was also used as a mono-therapy for different viral and bacterial infections. CpG 10101 (class C ODN) was tested in a Phase Ib trial for treating hepatitis C virus positive patients, where doses of up to 0.75 mg/kg were given weekly. The use of CPG 10101 caused a dose-dependent decrease in blood viral RNA levels, which was associated with biomarkers of TLR9 activation, like NK cell activation and serum IFN-α.

Although activation of the innate immune system could be demonstrated by cytokine and chemokine release, further studies are needed to demonstrate an adaptive immune response, including a virus-specific T cell response. CpG ODNs have been used as adjuvants for hepatitis B vaccination in at least two studies [144, 145].

In a randomized, double-blind Phase I dose escalation study, healthy volunteers were vaccinated at 0, 4 and 24 weeks by intramuscular injection with Engerix-B (GlaxoSmithKline) mixed with saline (control) or with CPG-7909. Anti-HBs appeared significantly sooner and were significantly higher in CPG-7909 recipients compared to control subjects, and most CPG-7909 vaccinated subjects developed protective levels of anti-HB IgG within just two weeks of the priming vaccine dose. A trend towards higher rates of positive cytotoxic T-cell lymphocyte responses was noted in the two higher dose groups of CPG-7909 compared to controls [145].

Table 3. TLR9 agonists in clinical use

CpG ODN	Class	Company	Uses
PF 3512676	B	Pfizer	Cancer monotherapy or in combination with other cancer therapies, vaccines
ODN CpG 10101	C	Coley	Hepatitis C virus Allergies, combination with monoclonal antibodies in cancer therapy, vaccines
ODN 1018 ISS	B	Dynavax	
IMO-2055		Idera	Cancer monotherapy Combination with chemotherapy

Conclusion

Our ability to dissect the immune response against pathogens, accompanied with advances in the field of molecular biology, have led to the introduction of more specific treatments that could substitute the old and crude way of using live attenuated pathogens, whole inactivated organisms, and inactivated toxins, for vaccines, which resulted in many undesirable side effects. Instead, recombinant proteins and synthetic peptides were used in newer vaccines, but they yielded poor immune responses due to their poor immunogenicity, unless combined with immunostimulatory adjuvants to induce a potent immune response.

Advances in our understanding of TLR functions enabled scientists to develop and use TLR agonists as vaccine adjuvants. In fact, many promising experimental vaccine strategies for both infectious diseases and for malignancies include the use of TLR ligands as adjuvants. Also, TLR agonists could be a very important asset in the development of non-antibiotic agents for the treatment of infection with multi-drug resistant pathogens. Moreover, our understanding of the downstream signaling of TLRs, and how they exert their functions could allow us to use reagents to enhance the signaling pathways, or modulate the TLR system to better fight infection or cancer.

References

[1] Seya T, Akazawa T, Tsujita T, Matsumoto M. Role of Toll-like receptors in adjuvant-augmented immune therapies. *Evid Based Complement Alternat Med.* 2006 Mar;3(1):31-8; discussion 133-7.

[2] Ishii KJ, Akira S. Toll or toll-free adjuvant path toward the optimal vaccine development. *Journal of clinical immunology.* 2007 Jul;27(4):363-71.

[3] Trinchieri G, Sher A. Cooperation of Toll-like receptor signals in innate immune defence. *Nature reviews.* 2007 Mar;7(3):179-90.

[4] Creagh EM, O'Neill LA. TLRs, NLRs and RLRs: a trinity of pathogen sensors that co-operate in innate immunity. *Trends in immunology.* 2006 Aug;27(8):352-7.

[5] Meylan E, Tschopp J, Karin M. Intracellular pattern recognition receptors in the host response. *Nature.* 2006 Jul 6;442(7098):39-44.

[6] Takeuchi O, Akira S. Signaling pathways activated by microorganisms. *Current opinion in cell biology.* 2007 Apr;19(2):185-91.

[7] Lemaitre B. The road to Toll. *Nature reviews.* 2004 Jul;4(7):521-7.

[8] Medzhitov R, Preston-Hurlburt P, Janeway CA, Jr. A human homologue of the Drosophila Toll protein signals activation of adaptive immunity. *Nature.* 1997 Jul 24;388(6640):394-7.

[9] van Duin D, Medzhitov R, Shaw AC. Triggering TLR signaling in vaccination. *Trends in immunology.* 2006 Jan;27(1):49-55.

[10] Bell JK, Mullen GE, Leifer CA, Mazzoni A, Davies DR, Segal DM. Leucine-rich repeats and pathogen recognition in Toll-like receptors. *Trends in immunology.* 2003 Oct;24(10):528-33.

[11] Janeway CA, Jr., Medzhitov R. Innate immune recognition. *Annual review of immunology.* 2002;20:197-216.

[12] Medzhitov R. Toll-like receptors and innate immunity. *Nature reviews.* 2001 Nov;1(2):135-45.

[13] Akira S. Toll-like receptors and innate immunity. *Advances in immunology.* 2001;78:1-56.

[14] Akira S, Takeda K. Toll-like receptor signalling. *Nature reviews.* 2004 Jul;4(7):499-511.

[15] Slack JL, Schooley K, Bonnert TP, Mitcham JL, Qwarnstrom EE, Sims JE, et al. Identification of two major sites in the type I interleukin-1 receptor cytoplasmic region

responsible for coupling to pro-inflammatory signaling pathways. *The Journal of biological chemistry.* 2000 Feb 18;275(7):4670-8.

[16] Wiemann B, Starnes CO. Coley's toxins, tumor necrosis factor and cancer research: a historical perspective. *Pharmacology and therapeutics.* 1994;64(3):529-64.

[17] Brightbill HD, Libraty DH, Krutzik SR, Yang RB, Belisle JT, Bleharski JR, et al. Host defense mechanisms triggered by microbial lipoproteins through toll-like receptors. *Science* (New York, NY. 1999 Jul 30;285(5428):732-6.

[18] West AP, Koblansky AA, Ghosh S. Recognition and signaling by toll-like receptors. *Annual review of cell and developmental biology.* 2006;22:409-37.

[19] O'Neill LA, Bowie AG. The family of five: TIR-domain-containing adaptors in Toll-like receptor signalling. *Nature reviews.* 2007 May;7(5):353-64.

[20] Yamamoto M, Sato S, Hemmi H, Hoshino K, Kaisho T, Sanjo H, et al. Role of adaptor TRIF in the MyD88-independent toll-like receptor signaling pathway. *Science* (New York, NY. 2003 Aug 1;301(5633):640-3.

[21] Hemmi H, Kaisho T, Takeuchi O, Sato S, Sanjo H, Hoshino K, et al. Small anti-viral compounds activate immune cells via the TLR7 MyD88-dependent signaling pathway. *Nature immunology.* 2002 Feb;3(2):196-200.

[22] Hoshino K, Kaisho T, Iwabe T, Takeuchi O, Akira S. Differential involvement of IFN-beta in Toll-like receptor-stimulated dendritic cell activation. *International immunology.* 2002 Oct;14(10):1225-31.

[23] Kawai T, Takeuchi O, Fujita T, Inoue J, Muhlradt PF, Sato S, et al. Lipopolysaccharide stimulates the MyD88-independent pathway and results in activation of IFN-regulatory factor 3 and the expression of a subset of lipopolysaccharide-inducible genes. *J. Immunol.* 2001 Nov 15;167(10):5887-94.

[24] [Horng T, Barton GM, Flavell RA, Medzhitov R. The adaptor molecule TIRAP provides signalling specificity for Toll-like receptors. *Nature.* 2002 Nov 21;420(6913):329-33.

[25] Yamamoto M, Sato S, Hemmi H, Sanjo H, Uematsu S, Kaisho T, et al. Essential role for TIRAP in activation of the signalling cascade shared by TLR2 and TLR4. *Nature.* 2002 Nov 21;420(6913):324-9.

[26] Yamamoto M, Sato S, Hemmi H, Uematsu S, Hoshino K, Kaisho T, et al. TRAM is specifically involved in the Toll-like receptor 4-mediated MyD88-independent signaling pathway. *Nature immunology.* 2003 Nov;4(11):1144-50.

[27] Chen ZJ. Ubiquitin signalling in the NF-kappaB pathway. *Nature cell biology.* 2005 Aug;7(8):758-65.

[28] Sato S, Sanjo H, Takeda K, Ninomiya-Tsuji J, Yamamoto M, Kawai T, et al. Essential function for the kinase TAK1 in innate and adaptive immune responses. *Nature immunology.* 2005 Nov;6(11):1087-95.

[29] Kawai T, Akira S. TLR signaling. *Seminars in immunology.* 2007 Feb;19(1):24-32.

[30] Kawai T, Adachi O, Ogawa T, Takeda K, Akira S. Unresponsiveness of MyD88-deficient mice to endotoxin. *Immunity.* 1999 Jul;11(1):115-22.

[31] Oshiumi H, Matsumoto M, Funami K, Akazawa T, Seya T. TICAM-1, an adaptor molecule that participates in Toll-like receptor 3-mediated interferon-beta induction. *Nature immunology.* 2003 Feb;4(2):161-7.

[32] Akira S, Uematsu S, Takeuchi O. Pathogen recognition and innate immunity. *Cell.* 2006 Feb 24;124(4):783-801.

[33] Hayden MS, West AP, Ghosh S. NF-kappaB and the immune response. *Oncogene.* 2006 Oct 30;25(51):6758-80.

[34] Hayden MS, West AP, Ghosh S. SnapShot: NF-kappaB signaling pathways. *Cell.* 2006 Dec 15;127(6):1286-7.

[35] Gilmore TD. Introduction to NF-kappaB: players, pathways, perspectives. *Oncogene.* 2006 Oct 30;25(51):6680-4.

[36] Kawai T, Akira S. Signaling to NF-kappaB by Toll-like receptors. *Trends in molecular medicine.* 2007 Nov;13(11):460-9.

[37] Tsuda Y, Takahashi H, Kobayashi M, Hanafusa T, Herndon DN, Suzuki F. Three different neutrophil subsets exhibited in mice with different susceptibilities to infection by methicillin-resistant Staphylococcus aureus. *Immunity.* 2004 Aug;21(2):215-26.

[38] Kurt-Jones EA, Mandell L, Whitney C, Padgett A, Gosselin K, Newburger PE, et al. Role of toll-like receptor 2 (TLR2) in neutrophil activation: GM-CSF enhances TLR2 expression and TLR2-mediated interleukin 8 responses in neutrophils. *Blood.* 2002 Sep 1;100(5):1860-8.

[39] Sabroe I, Jones EC, Usher LR, Whyte MK, Dower SK. Toll-like receptor (TLR)2 and TLR4 in human peripheral blood granulocytes: a critical role for monocytes in leukocyte lipopolysaccharide responses. *J. Immunol.* 2002 May 1;168(9):4701-10.

[40] Power CP, Wang JH, Manning B, Kell MR, Aherne NJ, Wu QD, et al. Bacterial lipoprotein delays apoptosis in human neutrophils through inhibition of caspase-3 activity: regulatory roles for CD14 and TLR-2. *J. Immunol.* 2004 Oct 15;173(8):5229-37.

[41] Francois S, El Benna J, Dang PM, Pedruzzi E, Gougerot-Pocidalo MA, Elbim C. Inhibition of neutrophil apoptosis by TLR agonists in whole blood: involvement of the phosphoinositide 3-kinase/Akt and NF-kappaB signaling pathways, leading to increased levels of Mcl-1, A1, and phosphorylated Bad. *J. Immunol.* 2005 Mar 15;174(6):3633-42.

[42] Remer KA, Brcic M, Jungi TW. Toll-like receptor-4 is involved in eliciting an LPS-induced oxidative burst in neutrophils. *Immunology letters.* 2003 Jan 2;85(1):75-80.

[43] Fan J, Malik AB. Toll-like receptor-4 (TLR4) signaling augments chemokine-induced neutrophil migration by modulating cell surface expression of chemokine receptors. *Nature medicine.* 2003 Mar;9(3):315-21.

[44] Sabroe I, Prince LR, Jones EC, Horsburgh MJ, Foster SJ, Vogel SN, et al. Selective roles for Toll-like receptor (TLR)2 and TLR4 in the regulation of neutrophil activation and life span. *J. Immunol.* 2003 May 15;170(10):5268-75.

[45] Sabroe I, Jones EC, Whyte MK, Dower SK. Regulation of human neutrophil chemokine receptor expression and function by activation of Toll-like receptors 2 and 4. *Immunology.* 2005 May;115(1):90-8.

[46] Hayashi F, Means TK, Luster AD. Toll-like receptors stimulate human neutrophil function. *Blood.* 2003 Oct 1;102(7):2660-9.

[47] Bozinovski S, Jones J, Beavitt SJ, Cook AD, Hamilton JA, Anderson GP. Innate immune responses to LPS in mouse lung are suppressed and reversed by neutralization

of GM-CSF via repression of TLR-4. *American journal of physiology.* 2004 Apr;286(4):L877-85.

[48] Ramphal R, Balloy V, Huerre M, Si-Tahar M, Chignard M. TLRs 2 and 4 are not involved in hypersusceptibility to acute Pseudomonas aeruginosa lung infections. *J. Immunol.* 2005 Sep 15;175(6):3927-34.

[49] Hajjar AM, Harowicz H, Liggitt HD, Fink PJ, Wilson CB, Skerrett SJ. An essential role for non-bone marrow-derived cells in control of Pseudomonas aeruginosa pneumonia. *Am. J. Respir. Cell Mol. Biol.* 2005 Nov;33(5):470-5.

[50] Shen XD, Ke B, Zhai Y, Gao F, Busuttil RW, Cheng G, et al. Toll-like receptor and heme oxygenase-1 signaling in hepatic ischemia/reperfusion injury. *Am. J. Transplant.* 2005 Aug;5(8):1793-800.

[51] Tsukamoto K, Hazeki K, Hoshi M, Nigorikawa K, Inoue N, Sasaki T, et al. Critical roles of the p110beta subtype of phosphoinositide 3-kinase in lipopolysaccharide-induced Akt activation and negative regulation of nitrite production in RAW 264.7 cells. *J. Immunol.* 2008 Feb 15;180(4):2054-61.

[52] Fukao T, Koyasu S. PI3K and negative regulation of TLR signaling. *Trends in immunology.* 2003 Jul;24(7):358-63.

[53] Guiducci C, Ghirelli C, Marloie-Provost MA, Matray T, Coffman RL, Liu YJ, et al. PI3K is critical for the nuclear translocation of IRF-7 and type I IFN production by human plasmacytoid predendritic cells in response to TLR activation. *The Journal of experimental medicine.* 2008 Feb 18;205(2):315-22.

[54] Schabbauer G, Luyendyk J, Crozat K, Jiang Z, Mackman N, Bahram S, et al. TLR4/CD14-mediated PI3K activation is an essential component of interferon-dependent VSV resistance in macrophages. *Molecular immunology.* 2008 Mar 11.

[55] Aksoy E, Vanden Berghe W, Detienne S, Amraoui Z, Fitzgerald KA, Haegeman G, et al. Inhibition of phosphoinositide 3-kinase enhances TRIF-dependent NF-kappa B activation and IFN-beta synthesis downstream of Toll-like receptor 3 and 4. *European journal of immunology.* 2005 Jul;35(7):2200-9.

[56] Yu Y, Nagai S, Wu H, Neish AS, Koyasu S, Gewirtz AT. TLR5-mediated phosphoinositide 3-kinase activation negatively regulates flagellin-induced proinflammatory gene expression. *J. Immunol.* 2006 May 15;176(10):6194-201.

[57] Rhee SH, Kim H, Moyer MP, Pothoulakis C. Role of MyD88 in phosphatidylinositol 3-kinase activation by flagellin/toll-like receptor 5 engagement in colonic epithelial cells. *The Journal of biological chemistry.* 2006 Jul 7;281(27):18560-8.

[58] Hazeki K, Kinoshita S, Matsumura T, Nigorikawa K, Kubo H, Hazeki O. Opposite effects of wortmannin and 2-(4-morpholinyl)-8-phenyl-1(4H)-benzopyran-4-one hydrochloride on toll-like receptor-mediated nitric oxide production: negative regulation of nuclear factor-{kappa}B by phosphoinositide 3-kinase. *Molecular pharmacology.* 2006 May;69(5):1717-24.

[59] Kuroda S, Nishio M, Sasaki T, Horie Y, Kawahara K, Sasaki M, et al. Effective clearance of intracellular Leishmania major in vivo requires Pten in macrophages. *European journal of immunology.* 2008 May;38(5):1331-40.

[60] Ha T, Hua F, Liu X, Ma J, McMullen JR, Shioi T, et al. Lipopolysaccharide-induced myocardial protection against ischaemia/reperfusion injury is mediated through a PI3K/Akt-dependent mechanism. *Cardiovascular research.* 2008 Mar 5.

[61] Arbibe L, Mira JP, Teusch N, Kline L, Guha M, Mackman N, et al. Toll-like receptor 2-mediated NF-kappa B activation requires a Rac1-dependent pathway. *Nature immunology.* 2000 Dec;1(6):533-40.

[62] Iwasaki A, Medzhitov R. Toll-like receptor control of the adaptive immune responses. *Nature immunology.* 2004 Oct;5(10):987-95.

[63] Schulz O, Diebold SS, Chen M, Naslund TI, Nolte MA, Alexopoulou L, et al. Toll-like receptor 3 promotes cross-priming to virus-infected cells. *Nature.* 2005 Feb 24;433(7028):887-92.

[64] Heit A, Schmitz F, O'Keeffe M, Staib C, Busch DH, Wagner H, et al. Protective CD8 T cell immunity triggered by CpG-protein conjugates competes with the efficacy of live vaccines. *J. Immunol.* 2005 Apr 1;174(7):4373-80.

[65] Spellberg B, Edwards JE, Jr. Type 1/Type 2 immunity in infectious diseases. *Clin. Infect. Dis.* 2001 Jan;32(1):76-102.

[66] Trinchieri G. Interleukin-12 and the regulation of innate resistance and adaptive immunity. *Nature reviews.* 2003 Feb;3(2):133-46.

[67] Gautier G, Humbert M, Deauvieau F, Scuiller M, Hiscott J, Bates EE, et al. A type I interferon autocrine-paracrine loop is involved in Toll-like receptor-induced interleukin-12p70 secretion by dendritic cells. *The Journal of experimental medicine.* 2005 May 2;201(9):1435-46.

[68] Pasare C, Medzhitov R. Toll pathway-dependent blockade of CD4+CD25+ T cell-mediated suppression by dendritic cells. Science (New York, NY. 2003 Feb 14;299(5609):1033-6.

[69] Yang Y, Huang CT, Huang X, Pardoll DM. Persistent Toll-like receptor signals are required for reversal of regulatory T cell-mediated CD8 tolerance. *Nature immunology.* 2004 May;5(5):508-15.

[70] Peng G, Guo Z, Kiniwa Y, Voo KS, Peng W, Fu T, et al. Toll-like receptor 8-mediated reversal of CD4+ regulatory T cell function. Science (New York, NY. 2005 Aug 26;309(5739):1380-4.

[71] Borst J, Hendriks J, Xiao Y. CD27 and CD70 in T cell and B cell activation. *Current opinion in immunology.* 2005 Jun;17(3):275-81.

[72] Diehl L, den Boer AT, Schoenberger SP, van der Voort EI, Schumacher TN, Melief CJ, et al. CD40 activation in vivo overcomes peptide-induced peripheral cytotoxic T-lymphocyte tolerance and augments anti-tumor vaccine efficacy. *Nature medicine.* 1999 Jul;5(7):774-9.

[73] Chen Z, Dehm S, Bonham K, Kamencic H, Juurlink B, Zhang X, et al. DNA array and biological characterization of the impact of the maturation status of mouse dendritic cells on their phenotype and antitumor vaccination efficacy. *Cellular immunology.* 2001 Nov 25;214(1):60-71.

[74] Hertz CJ, Kiertscher SM, Godowski PJ, Bouis DA, Norgard MV, Roth MD, et al. Microbial lipopeptides stimulate dendritic cell maturation via Toll-like receptor 2. *J. Immunol.* 2001 Feb 15;166(4):2444-50.

[75] Cella M, Engering A, Pinet V, Pieters J, Lanzavecchia A. Inflammatory stimuli induce accumulation of MHC class II complexes on dendritic cells. Nature. 1997 Aug 21;388(6644):782-7.

[76] Aliprantis AO, Yang RB, Mark MR, Suggett S, Devaux B, Radolf JD, et al. Cell activation and apoptosis by bacterial lipoproteins through toll-like receptor-2. Science (New York, NY. 1999 Jul 30;285(5428):736-9.

[77] Aliprantis AO, Yang RB, Weiss DS, Godowski P, Zychlinsky A. The apoptotic signaling pathway activated by Toll-like receptor-2. *The EMBO journal.* 2000 Jul 3;19(13):3325-36.

[78] Lien E, Sellati TJ, Yoshimura A, Flo TH, Rawadi G, Finberg RW, et al. Toll-like receptor 2 functions as a pattern recognition receptor for diverse bacterial products. The *Journal of biological chemistry.* 1999 Nov 19;274(47):33419-25.

[79] Schwandner R, Dziarski R, Wesche H, Rothe M, Kirschning CJ. Peptidoglycan- and lipoteichoic acid-induced cell activation is mediated by toll-like receptor 2. *The Journal of biological chemistry.* 1999 Jun 18;274(25):17406-9.

[80] Yoshimura A, Lien E, Ingalls RR, Tuomanen E, Dziarski R, Golenbock D. Cutting edge: recognition of Gram-positive bacterial cell wall components by the innate immune system occurs via Toll-like receptor 2. *J Immunol.* 1999 Jul 1;163(1):1-5.

[81] Underhill DM, Ozinsky A, Smith KD, Aderem A. Toll-like receptor-2 mediates mycobacteria-induced proinflammatory signaling in macrophages. Proceedings of the National Academy of Sciences of the United States of America. 1999 Dec 7;96(25):14459-63.

[82] Lehner MD, Morath S, Michelsen KS, Schumann RR, Hartung T. Induction of cross-tolerance by lipopolysaccharide and highly purified lipoteichoic acid via different Toll-like receptors independent of paracrine mediators. *J. Immunol.* 2001 Apr 15;166(8):5161-7.

[83] Means TK, Wang S, Lien E, Yoshimura A, Golenbock DT, Fenton MJ. Human toll-like receptors mediate cellular activation by Mycobacterium tuberculosis. *J. Immunol.* 1999 Oct 1;163(7):3920-7.

[84] Takeda K, Kaisho T, Akira S. Toll-like receptors. *Annual review of immunology.* 2003;21:335-76.

[85] Steere AC, Sikand VK, Meurice F, Parenti DL, Fikrig E, Schoen RT, et al. Vaccination against Lyme disease with recombinant Borrelia burgdorferi outer-surface lipoprotein A with adjuvant. Lyme Disease Vaccine Study Group. *The New England journal of medicine.* 1998 Jul 23;339(4):209-15.

[86] Alexopoulou L, Thomas V, Schnare M, Lobet Y, Anguita J, Schoen RT, et al. Hyporesponsiveness to vaccination with Borrelia burgdorferi OspA in humans and in TLR1- and TLR2-deficient mice. *Nature medicine.* 2002 Aug;8(8):878-84.

[87] Ozinsky A, Underhill DM, Fontenot JD, Hajjar AM, Smith KD, Wilson CB, et al. The repertoire for pattern recognition of pathogens by the innate immune system is defined by cooperation between toll-like receptors. Proceedings of the National Academy of Sciences of the United States of America. 2000 Dec 5;97(25):13766-71.

[88] Schneider C, Schmidt T, Ziske C, Tiemann K, Lee KM, Uhlinsky V, et al. Tumour suppression induced by the macrophage activating lipopeptide MALP-2 in an ultrasound guided pancreatic carcinoma mouse model. *Gut.* 2004 Mar;53(3):355-61.

[89] Beutler B, Jiang Z, Georgel P, Crozat K, Croker B, Rutschmann S, et al. Genetic analysis of host resistance: Toll-like receptor signaling and immunity at large. Annual review of immunology. 2006;24:353-89.

[90] da Silva Correia J, Soldau K, Christen U, Tobias PS, Ulevitch RJ. Lipopolysaccharide is in close proximity to each of the proteins in its membrane receptor complex. transfer from CD14 to TLR4 and MD-2. *The Journal of biological chemistry.* 2001 Jun 15;276(24):21129-35.

[91] da Silva Correia J, Ulevitch RJ. MD-2 and TLR4 N-linked glycosylations are important for a functional lipopolysaccharide receptor. *The Journal of biological chemistry.* 2002 Jan 18;277(3):1845-54.

[92] Galanos C, Luderitz O, Rietschel ET, Westphal O, Brade H, Brade L, et al. Synthetic and natural Escherichia coli free lipid A express identical endotoxic activities. *European journal of biochemistry / FEBS.* 1985 Apr 1;148(1):1-5.

[93] Takada H, Kotani S. Structural requirements of lipid A for endotoxicity and other biological activities. *Critical reviews in microbiology.* 1989;16(6):477-523.

[94] Takayama K, Qureshi N, Ribi E, Cantrell JL. Separation and characterization of toxic and nontoxic forms of lipid A. *Reviews of infectious diseases.* 1984 Jul-Aug;6(4):439-43.

[95] Qureshi N, Mascagni P, Ribi E, Takayama K. Monophosphoryl lipid A obtained from lipopolysaccharides of Salmonella minnesota R595. Purification of the dimethyl derivative by high performance liquid chromatography and complete structural determination. *The Journal of biological chemistry.* 1985 May 10;260(9):5271-8.

[96] Madonna GS, Peterson JE, Ribi EE, Vogel SN. Early-phase endotoxin tolerance: induction by a detoxified lipid A derivative, monophosphoryl lipid A. *Infection and immunity.* 1986 Apr;52(1):6-11.

[97] Thoelen S, Van Damme P, Mathei C, Leroux-Roels G, Desombere I, Safary A, et al. Safety and immunogenicity of a hepatitis B vaccine formulated with a novel adjuvant system. *Vaccine.* 1998 Apr;16(7):708-14.

[98] Stoute JA, Slaoui M, Heppner DG, Momin P, Kester KE, Desmons P, et al. A preliminary evaluation of a recombinant circumsporozoite protein vaccine against Plasmodium falciparum malaria. RTS,S Malaria Vaccine Evaluation Group. *The New England journal of medicine.* 1997 Jan 9;336(2):86-91.

[99] Takayama K, Ribi E, Cantrell JL. Isolation of a nontoxic lipid A fraction containing tumor regression activity. *Cancer research.* 1981 Jul;41(7):2654-7.

[100] Yang D, Satoh M, Ueda H, Tsukagoshi S, Yamazaki M. Activation of tumor-infiltrating macrophages by a synthetic lipid A analog (ONO-4007) and its implication in antitumor effects. *Cancer Immunol Immunother.* 1994 May;38(5):287-93.

[101] Kuramitsu Y, Nishibe M, Ohiro Y, Matsushita K, Yuan L, Obara M, et al. A new synthetic lipid A analog, ONO-4007, stimulates the production of tumor necrosis factor-alpha in tumor tissues, resulting in the rejection of transplanted rat hepatoma cells. *Anti-cancer drugs.* 1997 Jun;8(5):500-8.

[102] Garay RP, Viens P, Bauer J, Normier G, Bardou M, Jeannin JF, et al. Cancer relapse under chemotherapy: why TLR2/4 receptor agonists can help. *European journal of pharmacology*. 2007 Jun 1;563(1-3):1-17.

[103] Sato K, Yoo YC, Mochizuki M, Saiki I, Takahashi TA, Azuma I. Inhibition of tumor-induced angiogenesis by a synthetic lipid A analogue with low endotoxicity, DT-5461. *Jpn. J Cancer Res*. 1995 Apr;86(4):374-82.

[104] Kiani A, Tschiersch A, Gaboriau E, Otto F, Seiz A, Knopf HP, et al. Downregulation of the proinflammatory cytokine response to endotoxin by pretreatment with the nontoxic lipid A analog SDZ MRL 953 in cancer patients. *Blood*. 1997 Aug 15;90(4):1673-83.

[105] Hayashi F, Smith KD, Ozinsky A, Hawn TR, Yi EC, Goodlett DR, et al. The innate immune response to bacterial flagellin is mediated by Toll-like receptor 5. *Nature*. 2001 Apr 26;410(6832):1099-103.

[106] Eaves-Pyles T, Murthy K, Liaudet L, Virag L, Ross G, Soriano FG, et al. Flagellin, a novel mediator of Salmonella-induced epithelial activation and systemic inflammation: I kappa B alpha degradation, induction of nitric oxide synthase, induction of proinflammatory mediators, and cardiovascular dysfunction. *J. Immunol*. 2001 Jan 15;166(2):1248-60.

[107] Eaves-Pyles TD, Wong HR, Odoms K, Pyles RB. Salmonella flagellin-dependent proinflammatory responses are localized to the conserved amino and carboxyl regions of the protein. *J. Immunol*. 2001 Dec 15;167(12):7009-16.

[108] Murthy KG, Deb A, Goonesekera S, Szabo C, Salzman AL. Identification of conserved domains in Salmonella muenchen flagellin that are essential for its ability to activate TLR5 and to induce an inflammatory response in vitro. *The Journal of biological chemistry*. 2004 Feb 13;279(7):5667-75.

[109] Burdelya LG, Krivokrysenko VI, Tallant TC, Strom E, Gleiberman AS, Gupta D, et al. An agonist of toll-like receptor 5 has radioprotective activity in mouse and primate models. Science (New York, NY. 2008 Apr 11;320(5873):226-30.

[110] McDonald WF, Huleatt JW, Foellmer HG, Hewitt D, Tang J, Desai P, et al. A West Nile virus recombinant protein vaccine that coactivates innate and adaptive immunity. *The Journal of infectious diseases*. 2007 Jun 1;195(11):1607-17.

[111] Huleatt JW, Jacobs AR, Tang J, Desai P, Kopp EB, Huang Y, et al. Vaccination with recombinant fusion proteins incorporating Toll-like receptor ligands induces rapid cellular and humoral immunity. *Vaccine*. 2007 Jan 8;25(4):763-75.

[112] Huleatt JW, Nakaar V, Desai P, Huang Y, Hewitt D, Jacobs A, et al. Potent immunogenicity and efficacy of a universal influenza vaccine candidate comprising a recombinant fusion protein linking influenza M2e to the TLR5 ligand flagellin. *Vaccine*. 2008 Jan 10;26(2):201-14.

[113] Gorden KB, Gorski KS, Gibson SJ, Kedl RM, Kieper WC, Qiu X, et al. Synthetic TLR agonists reveal functional differences between human TLR7 and TLR8. *J. Immunol*. 2005 Feb 1;174(3):1259-68.

[114] Triantafilou K, Vakakis E, Orthopoulos G, Ahmed MA, Schumann C, Lepper PM, et al. TLR8 and TLR7 are involved in the host's immune response to human parechovirus 1. *European journal of immunology*. 2005 Aug;35(8):2416-23.

[115] Triantafilou K, Orthopoulos G, Vakakis E, Ahmed MA, Golenbock DT, Lepper PM, et al. Human cardiac inflammatory responses triggered by Coxsackie B viruses are mainly Toll-like receptor (TLR) 8-dependent. *Cell Microbiol.* 2005 Aug;7(8):1117-26.

[116] Sioud M, Floisand Y, Forfang L, Lund-Johansen F. Signaling through toll-like receptor 7/8 induces the differentiation of human bone marrow CD34+ progenitor cells along the myeloid lineage. *Journal of molecular biology.* 2006 Dec 15;364(5):945-54.

[117] Garantziotis S, Hollingsworth JW, Zaas AK, Schwartz DA. The effect of toll-like receptors and toll-like receptor genetics in human disease. *Annual review of medicine.* 2008;59:343-59.

[118] Zhu J, Lai K, Brownile R, Babiuk LA, Mutwiri GK. Porcine TLR8 and TLR7 are both activated by a selective TLR7 ligand, imiquimod. *Molecular immunology.* 2008 Jun;45(11):3238-43.

[119] Craft N, Bruhn KW, Nguyen BD, Prins R, Lin JW, Liau LM, et al. The TLR7 agonist imiquimod enhances the anti-melanoma effects of a recombinant Listeria monocytogenes vaccine. *J. Immunol.* 2005 Aug 1;175(3):1983-90.

[120] Stary G, Bangert C, Tauber M, Strohal R, Kopp T, Stingl G. Tumoricidal activity of TLR7/8-activated inflammatory dendritic cells. *The Journal of experimental medicine.* 2007 Jun 11;204(6):1441-51.

[121] Redondo P, del Olmo J, Lopez-Diaz de Cerio A, Inoges S, Marquina M, Melero I, et al. Imiquimod enhances the systemic immunity attained by local cryosurgery destruction of melanoma lesions. *The Journal of investigative dermatology.* 2007 Jul;127(7):1673-80.

[122] Horsmans Y, Berg T, Desager JP, Mueller T, Schott E, Fletcher SP, et al. Isatoribine, an agonist of TLR7, reduces plasma virus concentration in chronic hepatitis C infection. *Hepatology* (Baltimore, Md. 2005 Sep;42(3):724-31.

[123] Deane JA, Pisitkun P, Barrett RS, Feigenbaum L, Town T, Ward JM, et al. Control of toll-like receptor 7 expression is essential to restrict autoimmunity and dendritic cell proliferation. *Immunity.* 2007 Nov;27(5):801-10.

[124] Barrat FJ, Meeker T, Chan JH, Guiducci C, Coffman RL. Treatment of lupus-prone mice with a dual inhibitor of TLR7 and TLR9 leads to reduction of autoantibody production and amelioration of disease symptoms. *European journal of immunology.* 2007 Dec;37(12):3582-6.

[125] Dudek AZ, Yunis C, Harrison LI, Kumar S, Hawkinson R, Cooley S, et al. First in human phase I trial of 852A, a novel systemic toll-like receptor 7 agonist, to activate innate immune responses in patients with advanced cancer. *Clin. Cancer Res.* 2007 Dec 1;13(23):7119-25.

[126] Dummer R, Hauschild A, Becker JC, Grob JJ, Schadendorf D, Tebbs V, et al. An exploratory study of systemic administration of the toll-like receptor-7 agonist 852A in patients with refractory metastatic melanoma. *Clin. Cancer Res.* 2008 Feb 1;14(3):856-64.

[127] Moisan J, Camateros P, Thuraisingam T, Marion D, Koohsari H, Martin P, et al. TLR7 ligand prevents allergen-induced airway hyperresponsiveness and eosinophilia in allergic asthma by a MYD88-dependent and MK2-independent pathway. *American journal of physiology.* 2006 May;290(5):L987-95.

[128] Camateros P, Tamaoka M, Hassan M, Marino R, Moisan J, Marion D, et al. Chronic asthma-induced airway remodeling is prevented by toll-like receptor-7/8 ligand S28463. *American journal of respiratory and critical care medicine.* 2007 Jun 15;175(12):1241-9.

[129] Hammerbeck DM, Burleson GR, Schuller CJ, Vasilakos JP, Tomai M, Egging E, et al. Administration of a dual toll-like receptor 7 and toll-like receptor 8 agonist protects against influenza in rats. *Antiviral research.* 2007 Jan;73(1):1-11.

[130] Leifer CA, Kennedy MN, Mazzoni A, Lee C, Kruhlak MJ, Segal DM. TLR9 is localized in the endoplasmic reticulum prior to stimulation. *J. Immunol.* 2004 Jul 15;173(2):1179-83.

[131] Latz E, Schoenemeyer A, Visintin A, Fitzgerald KA, Monks BG, Knetter CF, et al. TLR9 signals after translocating from the ER to CpG DNA in the lysosome. *Nature immunology.* 2004 Feb;5(2):190-8.

[132] Ahmad-Nejad P, Hacker H, Rutz M, Bauer S, Vabulas RM, Wagner H. Bacterial CpG-DNA and lipopolysaccharides activate Toll-like receptors at distinct cellular compartments. *European journal of immunology.* 2002 Jul;32(7):1958-68.

[133] Faith A, Peek E, McDonald J, Urry Z, Richards DF, Tan C, et al. Plasmacytoid dendritic cells from human lung cancer draining lymph nodes induce Tc1 responses. *Am.. J. Respir. Cell Mol. Biol.* 2007 Mar;36(3):360-7.

[134] Bernasconi NL, Onai N, Lanzavecchia A. A role for Toll-like receptors in acquired immunity: up-regulation of TLR9 by BCR triggering in naive B cells and constitutive expression in memory B cells. *Blood.* 2003 Jun 1;101(11):4500-4.

[135] Krieg AM. Therapeutic potential of Toll-like receptor 9 activation. *Nature reviews.* 2006 Jun;5(6):471-84.

[136] Krug A, Rothenfusser S, Selinger S, Bock C, Kerkmann M, Battiany J, et al. CpG-A oligonucleotides induce a monocyte-derived dendritic cell-like phenotype that preferentially activates CD8 T cells. *J. Immunol.* 2003 Apr 1;170(7):3468-77.

[137] Kerkmann M, Costa LT, Richter C, Rothenfusser S, Battiany J, Hornung V, et al. Spontaneous formation of nucleic acid-based nanoparticles is responsible for high interferon-alpha induction by CpG-A in plasmacytoid dendritic cells. *The Journal of biological chemistry.* 2005 Mar 4;280(9):8086-93.

[138] Hartmann G, Battiany J, Poeck H, Wagner M, Kerkmann M, Lubenow N, et al. Rational design of new CpG oligonucleotides that combine B cell activation with high IFN-alpha induction in plasmacytoid dendritic cells. *European journal of immunology.* 2003 Jun;33(6):1633-41.

[139] Krieg AM. CpG motifs in bacterial DNA and their immune effects. *Annual review of immunology.* 2002;20:709-60.

[140] Murad YM, Clay TM, Lyerly HK, Morse MA. CPG-7909 (PF-3512676, ProMune): toll-like receptor-9 agonist in cancer therapy. *Expert opinion on biological therapy.* 2007 Aug;7(8):1257-66.

[141] Krieg AM. Development of TLR9 agonists for cancer therapy. The Journal of clinical investigation. 2007 May;117(5):1184-94.

[142] Hayashi T, Raz E. TLR9-based immunotherapy for allergic disease. *The American journal of medicine.* 2006 Oct;119(10):897 e1-6.

[143] Creticos PS, Schroeder JT, Hamilton RG, Balcer-Whaley SL, Khattignavong AP, Lindblad R, et al. Immunotherapy with a ragweed-toll-like receptor 9 agonist vaccine for allergic rhinitis. *The New England journal of medicine.* 2006 Oct 5;355(14):1445-55.

[144] Halperin SA, Van Nest G, Smith B, Abtahi S, Whiley H, Eiden JJ. A phase I study of the safety and immunogenicity of recombinant hepatitis B surface antigen co-administered with an immunostimulatory phosphorothioate oligonucleotide adjuvant. *Vaccine.* 2003 Jun 2;21(19-20):2461-7.

[145] Cooper CL, Davis HL, Morris ML, Efler SM, Adhami MA, Krieg AM, et al. CPG 7909, an immunostimulatory TLR9 agonist oligodeoxynucleotide, as adjuvant to Engerix-B HBV vaccine in healthy adults: a double-blind phase I/II study. *Journal of clinical immunology.* 2004 Nov;24(6):693-701.

Chapter 3

Modulating Immune Response with CpG-Oligodeoxynucleotide through the Skin

Joe Inoue[1] and Yukihiko Aramaki[2]

1. Department of Biosciences, School of Science and Graduate School of Science, Kitasato University, Japan
2. School of Pharmacy, Tokyo University of Pharmacy and Life Sciences, Japan

Abstract

Unmethylated CpG dinucleotides flanked by certain bases (CpG-motif), which are present in bacterial DNA, have been shown to be immunostimulatory. Previous studies have found that both bacterial CpG-motifs and synthetic oligodeoxynucleotides containing a CpG-motif (CpG-ODN) activate cells such as B-cells, macrophages and dendritic cells (DC), through toll-like receptor-9 (TLR-9). Signaling through TLR-9 has been shown to lead to the secretion of large amounts of cytokines such as type-I IFN and IL-12. These cytokines act on T cells inducing the production of cytokines, primarily IFN-γ. CpG-ODN also induces the production of great numbers of CTLs which have anti-tumor effects. Consequently, CpG-ODN could be effective as an adjuvant for humoral and cellular immunities.

We have demonstrated that the administration of CpG-ODN through the skin induced a Th1-type immune response and this suggests that the skin is a potential site for vaccination. Additionally, the transcutaneous vaccination of a tumor-antigen and CpG-ODN in combination with a COX-2 inhibitor was effective in inducing antigen-specific anti-tumor immunity *in vivo*. These results suggest that this transcutaneous vaccination is an effective approach for the development of tumor vaccines.

We have also reported that administration of CpG-ODN through the skin may shift the immune response from type Th2 to Th1 and drastically attenuate the production of IgE in mice undergoing an IgE-type immune response. The application of CpG-ODN remarkably changed the immune response from type Th2 to Th1 in NC/Nga mice which spontaneously developed atopic dermatitis (AD)-like symptoms and high-Th2-immune responses. These results suggest CpG-ODN is effective for immunotherapy in patients with AD, which is characterized by Th2-dominated inflammation.

In summary, vaccination with CpG-ODN through the skin is a very simple and cost effective strategy for the development of tumor vaccine and immunotherapy in patients with AD and may be readily achievable.

Introduction

Vaccinations are one of the most cost-effective ways to prevent and control diseases and there is still a great need to develop a new generation of safer vaccines that can be effectively administered by simple, economical, and practical immunization procedures. Recently, there has been a lot of interest in the potential of non-invasive routes, such as via the skin, for vaccine delivery [1-8]. This recent interest is because skin-associated lymphoid tissue, comprised of powerful antigen-presenting cells (APCs), such as Langerhans cells (LCs), dermal dendritic cells (DCs), re-circulating T cells, and regional LNs, ensures the efficient presentation of antigens to immunocompetent cells and induction of strong immune responses. In addition, LCs and dermal DCs commonly exist in the skin and are easy to target [9].

Unmethylated CpG dinucleotides flanked by certain bases (CpG-motif), which are present in bacterial DNA, have been shown to be immunostimulatory [10]. Previous studies have found that both bacterial CpG-motifs and synthetic oligodeoxynucleotides containing a CpG-motif (CpG-ODN) activate cells such as B-cells, macrophages, and dendritic cells (DC), through toll-like receptor-9 (TLR-9) [10, 11]. Signaling through TLR-9 has been shown to lead to the secretion of large amounts of pro-inflammatory cytokines such as type-I IFN, IL-1β, IL-6, TNF-α, and IL-12 [12, 13]. IL-12 acts on T and NK cells inducing the production of cytokines, primarily IFN-γ, enhancing NK cell cytotoxic activity. CpG-ODN also induces the production of great numbers of cytotoxic T lymphocytes (CTLs) which have anti-tumor effects [14, 15]. Consequently, CpG-ODN could be effective as an adjuvant for humoral and cellular immunities [16].

CD4$^+$ helper T (Th) cells are subdivided into at least two subsets, Th1 and Th2, on the basis of the cytokines they secrete [17,18]. Th1-like immune responses enhance cellular immunity in association with increased levels of Th1-like cytokines such as IL-2 and IFN-γ and up-regulated activity of CTLs, indicating that the suppression of Th1 cells and CTLs can result in an acceleration of tumor growth [19]. One of the principal goals in tumor immune prophylaxis and tumor therapy is the induction of anti-tumor responses by generating sufficient numbers of tumor antigen-specific Th1 cells and CTLs.

Dysregulated Th1 or Th2 responses are also thought to be central to the pathology of diseases such as AD and asthma, which are characterized by Th2-dominated allergic inflammation [20-22]. Th2-like immune responses mediated by IL-4, IL-5 and IL-13 are keys to the pathogenesis of atopic disorders, because the up-regulation of IgE production, one of the major causes of atopic inflammation, has been extensively regulated with Th2 cytokines, IL-4 and IL-13. Th2 cell numbers increase in the lesional tissues of patients who suffer from atopic diseases and patients with AD frequently show elevated IgE levels in response to many kinds of allergens such as mite antigens and house dust [23, 24]. Therefore, it is very important to consider the balance of Th1 and Th2 in patients with immune diseases especially in allergic diseases.

We have demonstrated that the administration of CpG-ODN through the skin induced a Th1-type immune response and this suggests that the skin is a potential site for vaccination. We have also reported that administration of CpG-ODN through the skin may shift the immune response from type Th2 to Th1 and drastically attenuate the production of IgE in mice undergoing an IgE-type immune response. Thus, it is a straightforward strategy to use CpG-ODN which induces a Th1-type immune response, for tumor vaccination and immunotherapy for patients with diseases like AD that are associated with a Th2-predominant immune response. The present review focuses on the modulating immune response with CpG-ODN through the skin in mice.

The Skin

The skin is the largest organ of the body [25], accounting for more than 10% of body mass, and the one that enables the body to interact more intimately with its environment. Essentially, the skin consists of four layers (Figure 1): The stratum corneum, that is the outer layer of the skin, and forms the rate-controlling barrier for diffusion for almost all compounds. The other layers are the epidermis, the dermis, and subcutaneous tissue.

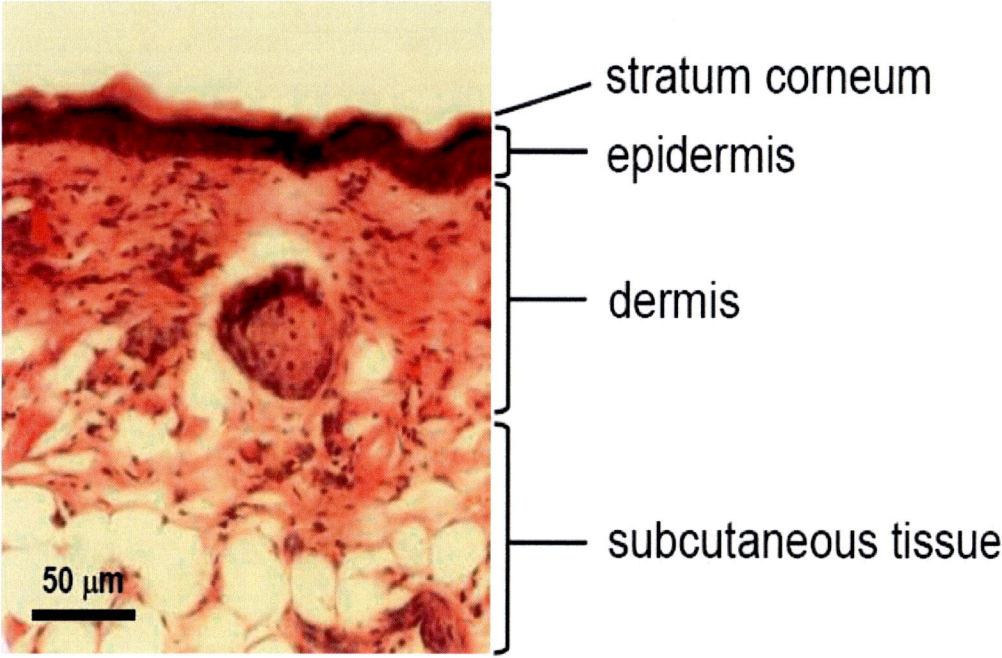

Figure 1. Layers of mouse skin: HE staining.

The skin has recently become a target site in the development of non-invasive vaccine technologies. It is also favorable that APCs, especially Langerhans cells (LCs) and dermal DCs, are common in the skin and easy to target. Thus, the skin is one of the most potential sites for vaccination.

Vaccination through the Skin

We used a tape-stripping technique for vaccination (Figure 2). This technique is the simplest method for reducing the barrier imposed by the stratum corneum. In detail, mice were anesthetized and square 20 mm of the abdominal skin was shaved with a disposal razor, and then the stratum corneum was removed by stripping with adhesive tape for 6-10 times.

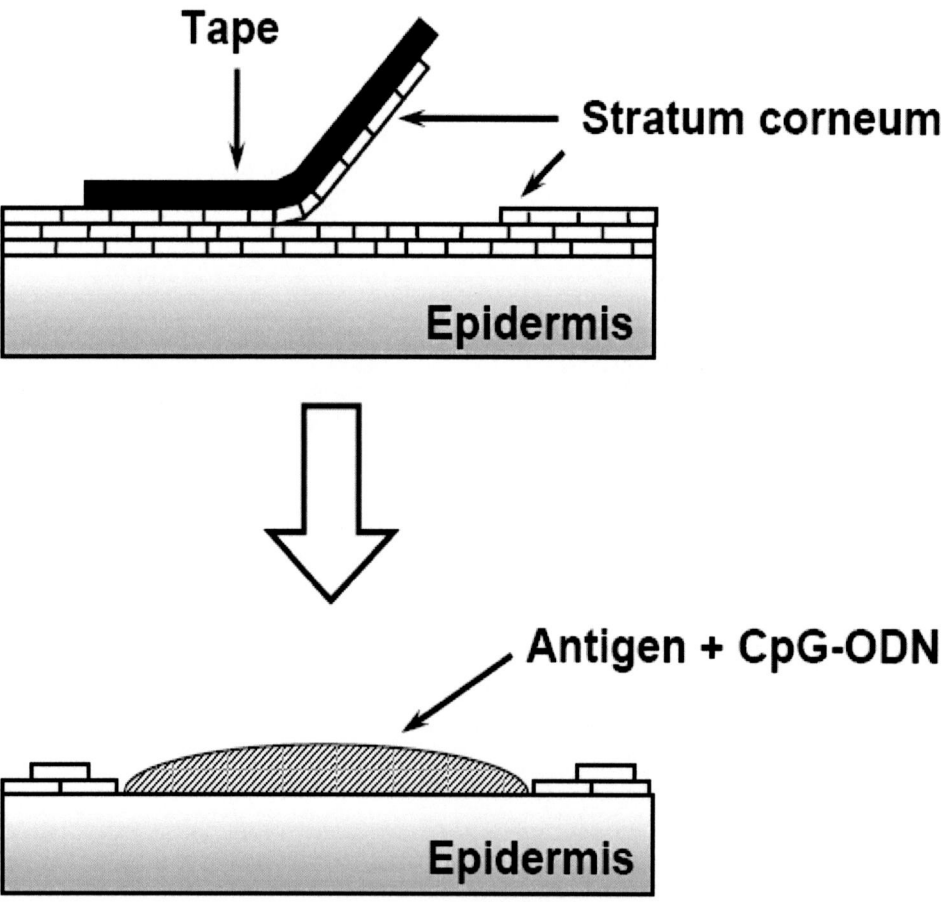

Figure 2 Method of tape-stripping.

Then, we examined the localization of the antigen and CpG-ODN following the application to tape-stripped skin. Since tape-stripping is a simple way to remove the epidermal barrier of the stratum corneum [26], the model antigen, ovalbumin (OVA) with a molecular weight of 45,000, and CpG-ODN, having high water solubility, easily penetrated the skin [27, 28]. However, no absorption of the antigen and CpG-ODN was observed from normal skin, and these compounds were trapped in the stratum corneum. Co-administration of CpG-ODN and OVA to tape-stripped skin elicited an antigen-specific Th1-predominant immune response and enhanced the production of Th1-type cytokines, IL-12 and IFN-γ. On the other hand, the production of a Th2-type cytokine, IL-4, was drastically suppressed. In terms of antigen-specific antibody production, the level of IgG2a, which is regulated by IFN-γ, was increased by CpG-ODN, but IgE production regulated by IL-4 was suppressed [27-29]. Additionally, we demonstrated that tape-stripping induces the expression of toll-like receptor (TLR)-9 in the skin, and enhances the Th1-type immune response triggered by CpG-ODN administered through the tape-stripped skin [30].

The transdermal application of CpG-ODN with an antigen through the tape-stripped skin is an effective way to induce a Th1-type immune response, and is also a simple, cost-effective, and needle-free vaccination system. Additionally, transcutaneous vaccination with tape-stripping was effective in human [31], therefore the skin is an attractive target for vaccine delivery in human too.

For Tumor Vaccines

Recently, there has been a lot of interest in the potential of non-invasive routes, such as via the skin, for tumor vaccine delivery [1-5]. Because skin-associated lymphoid tissue, comprised of powerful APCs such as LCs and dermal DCs, re-circulating T cells, and regional LNs, ensures the efficient presentation of tumor antigen to immunocompetent cells and induction of strong immune responses. We have recently reported that the administration of CpG-ODN through tape-stripped skin induced an antigen-specific Th1-type immune response and suggested that the skin is a potential site for vaccination [27-30]. However, it could not induce sufficient immunities for tumor therapy. Therefore, we tried to establish efficient Th1 and CTL priming strategies against tumors, using a COX-2 inhibitor and CpG-ODN applied to the skin [32].

Cyclooxygenase (COX)-2 and its product prostaglandin (PG) E_2 underlie an immunosuppressive network that is important in tumor therapy and vaccination [33, 34]. CpG-ODN induces pro-inflammatory cytokines such as type-I IFN and IL-12 which induces CTLs and Th1, CpG-ODN induces COX-2 expression and PGE_2 production in DCs and macrophages as well [35, 36]. PGE_2 is a potent inhibitor of Th1-type immune responses [37], inhibiting IFN-γ production as well as IL-12 and IL-12R expression [38, 39], and is also a potent inducer of production of the immunosuppressive cytokine IL-10 [40]. Furthermore, IL-10 suppresses the production of IL-12 by antigen-presenting cells (APCs), therefore APCs from IL-10 knockout mice were induced to produce a large quantity of IL-12 by CpG-ODN [41]. Thus, it is very simple strategy to use a COX-2 inhibitor for tumor vaccination with CpG-ODN.

First, we examined whether the COX-2 inhibitor NS-398, enhances the antigen-specific Th1-dominant immune response induced by CpG-ODN, applied to tape-stripped skin in mice. The production of IFN-γ increased on the co-application of OVA and CpG-ODN, and up-regulation of IFN-γ production was observed in mice treated with the COX-2 inhibitor. Next, we examined the production of OVA-specific IgG2a antibody which is considered to be a Th1-like Ig isotype. OVA-specific IgG2a production increased drastically when NS-398 was applied with CpG-ODN from the skin. These findings suggest that co-application of CpG-ODN with a COX-2 inhibitor to tape-stripped skin leads to enhanced Th1-dominant immune responses.

What is the enhancement mechanism of Th1-type immune responses induced by the transcutaneous vaccination with a COX-2 inhibitor? It has been reported that CpG-ODN promotes Th1-like immune responses with the production of PGE_2 and IL-10, which are considered to be suppressive mediators *in vivo*. As such, we first examined the changes in cytokine levels in the skin after transcutaneous vaccination. IL-12, IL-10, and PGE_2 levels increased significantly when OVA was co-applied with CpG-ODN. On the other hand, the application of NS-398 drastically increased IL-12 production but significantly decreased IL-10 and PGE_2 production in the skin. These findings suggest that NS-398 suppresses the production of PGE_2 and IL-10 in the skin and this suppression induces the production of a large quantity of IL-12.

It has been reported that the number of allergen-bearing LCs in the LN was significantly greater in IL-10 knockout mice than in wild-type mice, and these mice demonstrated a greater increase in the production of TNF-α and IL-1β, which induce the migration of LCs to the LN in allergen-exposed epidermis [42]. So, we next examined the effect of a COX-2 inhibitor on the migration of APCs to draining LNs. NS-398, CpG-ODN, and Alexa-488-conjugated OVA were applied to tape-stripped skin, and the draining LNs were removed. LN single cells were treated with anti-MHC class II mAb or anti-CD11c mAb and then double-positive cells were analyzed by FACScan. The application of CpG-ODN to the tape-stripped skin significantly enhanced the migration of Alexa-488 and MHC class II double positive cells, but any significant differences between CpG-ODN and CpG-ODN plus NS-398 were not observed. In the case of CD11c analysis, the migration of Alexa-488 and CD11c double positive cells to draining LNs were significantly enhanced when NS-398 was co-applied. These results suggest that the co-application with NS-398 especially enhances the migration of antigen-bearing-CD11c positive cells to the draining LNs.

Therefore, we next examined the effect of these APCs on T cell differentiation in the draining LN. NS-398, CpG-ODN, and OVA were applied to the tape-stripped skin, then draining LNs were removed, and the cytokine mRNA expression in the LN was determined by RT-PCR. The expression of IL-10 mRNA induced by CpG-ODN treatment was clearly reduced by NS-398. On the other hand, IL-12 mRNA was clearly expressed in the LNs of NS-398-treated mice. These findings suggest that the migration of LCs and dermal DCs, which acquired the ability to produce IL-12 by NS-398 and CpG-ODN treatment, or direct delivery of these drugs induces a high expression of IFN-γ mRNA in the draining LN. It has also been reported that IL-12 induces Th1 differentiation [43, 44], and our experiment shows that the IFN-γ mRNA expression induced mainly by Th1 in the LN was up-regulated with the application of NS-398.

Next, we examined whether the COX-2 inhibitor NS-398 enhances the generation and activity of CTLs induced by CpG-ODN. NS-398, OVA and CpG-ODN were applied to the skin, and spleen cells were prepared on seven days after the vaccination. To generate CTLs, spleen cells were stimulated with Mitomycin C-treated E.G7-OVA cells (transfected with EL4 to express OVA) and cultured for five days. Then, CTLs and E.G7-OVA cells were incubated. Specific cell lysis was observed in spleen cells prepared from CpG-ODN-treated mice and this CTL activity was significantly increased in CpG-ODN plus NS-398-treated mice. Thus, NS-398 enhances not only Th1-type immune responses but also CTL activities.

It is very important for tumor immune prophylaxis and tumor therapy to induce anti-tumor responses by generating sufficient numbers of tumor antigen-specific Th1 cells and CTLs. We examined the effect of a COX-2 inhibitor on the generation of antigen-specific Th1 cells and CTLs by CpG-ODN and showed that vaccination with such an inhibitor from the skin increased the numbers and activity of these cells. Subsequently, we examined tumor immune prophylaxis on transcutaneous vaccination with the COX-2 inhibitor. Following transcutaneous vaccination, mice were inoculated s.c. with E.G7-OVA tumor cells, and subsequent tumor growth was assessed by measuring tumor volume. Tumor growth was inhibited in CpG-ODN-treated mice and this inhibitory effect was significantly enhanced when mice were treated with NS-398. Furthermore, 60% of NS-398-treated mice survived 100 days, but only 10% of the mice treated with only CpG-ODN survived.

All these findings suggest that transcutaneous vaccination with a COX-2 inhibitor is a very simple and effective way to induce anti-tumor immunity and that such a vaccine is both non-invasive and effective (Figure 3). In addition, COX-2 inhibitors are commonly used in clinical medicines, therefore this strategy should be readily achievable when the use of CpG-ODN is authorized.

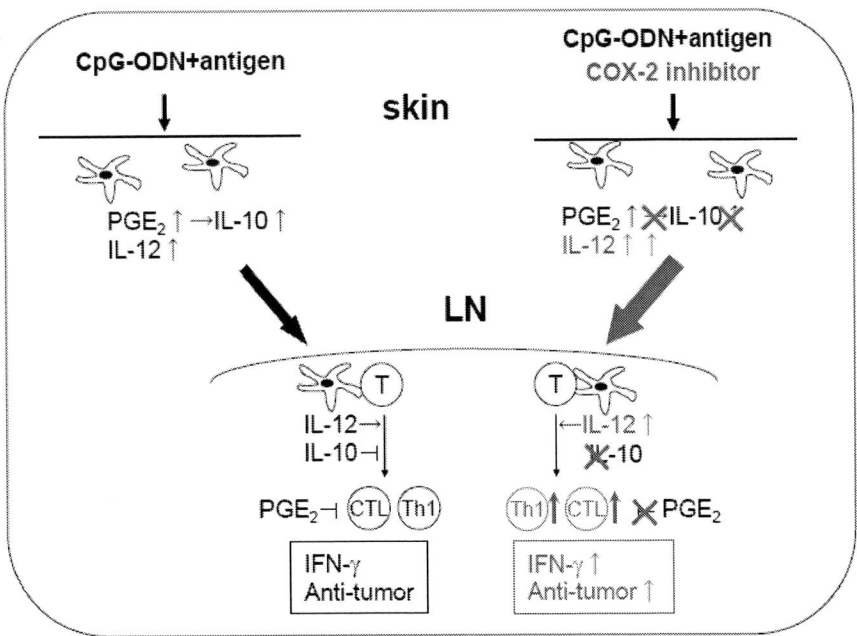

Figure 3. Mechanism of transcutaneous vaccination with COX-2 inhibitor.

For Atopic Disorders

Atopic disorders (AD) have a complex and chronic pathogenesis that provides many potential cellular and molecular targets for therapeutic intervention, but may also include redundant pathways mediating disease [45, 46]. In AD, skin lesions show a chronically relapsing inflammatory disorder with prurience and eczema usually associated with elevated serum IgE levels [47, 48]. The skin lesions of AD patients are characterized by the presence of inflammatory infiltrates consisting of T lymphocytes, monocytes/macrophages, eosinophils, and mast cells [49, 50].

NC/Nga mice are an inbred strain established from Japanese fancy mice in 1957 by Kondo (Nagoya University, Nagoya, Japan) [51]. When kept under conventional (CONV) conditions, they start to scratch themselves at about eight weeks, and their skin becomes dry and scaly. Within the next several weeks, the mice develop lesions on the ears, back, neck, and face. Immunohistochemical examination of the lesions in CONV NC/Nga mice reveal hyperkeratosis, acanthosis, and parakeratosis, all of which resemble the typical features of the skin observed in patients with AD [52]. The lesions show lymphocyte and macrophage infiltration, as well as mast cell and eosinophil degranulation. In addition, the level of IgE in the serum gradually increases [53]. All these immunological, histological, and biochemical changes in CONV NC/Nga mice resemble human AD. In fact, our examination showed that, in CONV NC/Nga mice, serum IgE levels were extremely high and mRNA levels of Th2-type cytokines and chemokines in the draining lymph node (LN) were expressed but not in IFN-γ, which is classified as a Th1-type cytokine [54]. From these findings, we confirmed that the CONV NC/Nga mice used in this experiment show high-Th2-like immune responses and the up-regulation of IgE production regulated by Th2 cytokines, IL-4 and IL-13, is one of the major causes of atopic inflammation.

In AD patients, a deficiency in the barrier function of the skin at the lesional site was reported [55]. Therefore, environmental allergens such as mites and house dust easily penetrate such susceptible skin. So, we first examined the penetration of CpG-ODN by the barrier-disrupted AD skin in CONV NC/Nga mice. Rhodamine-labeled CpG-ODN (Rho-CpG-ODN) was applied to the shaved back and its localization was examined by confocal laser scanning microscopy. In the skin of NC/Nga mice kept under SPF conditions, fluorescent signals for Rhodamine were observed faintly in the stratum corneum, suggesting that CpG-ODN didn't penetrate the subcutaneous layer. In the CONV NC/Nga mice, however, red-fluorescence generated from Rhodamine was observed around the corium after application, indicating that CpG-ODN has a molecular weight of more than 6,000 and a negative charge and easily penetrated the skin. From these findings, the barrier function of CONV NC/Nga mouse skin was disrupted as in AD patients.

We next examined the effect of CpG-ODN on the production of antibodies. To examine the changes in antibody levels, 50 μg of CpG-ODN or non-CpG-ODN was applied to the skin lesions every week eight times from week 11, which is when they first developed. Total IgE levels decreased from 24 weeks and a significant difference from the control and non-CpG-ODN was observed at 28-33 weeks. On the other hand, IgG2a levels increased significantly at 20-24 weeks in mice applied CpG-ODN. The total amount of IgG1, which is characterized as a Th2-type antibody, decreased drastically as did the profile of IgE production. These results indicated that the application of CpG-ODN changes the immune responses in CONV NC/Nga mice which show a Th2-predominant reaction.

Next, we examined the changes in mRNA levels of cytokines and chemokines in the draining lymph node (LN) at 33 weeks, because production of IgE decreased significantly compared to the control at that time. The mRNA levels of the Th2-type cytokines and chemokines were decreased in the CpG-ODN-treated NC/Nga mice. On the other hand, the mRNA levels of Th1-type cytokines, IFN-γ and IL-12, increased slightly in the CpG-ODN-treated NC/Nga mice. The mRNA levels of TNF-α and chemokines, both inflammatory markers, decreased in the CpG-ODN-treated mice. These findings suggest that transdermal application of CpG-ODN changes the immune response of NC/Nga, which is predominantly type Th2. Decreases in IL-4 and IL-13 mRNA expressions in the CpG-ODN-treated mice could result in suppression in IgE production. Interestingly, CpG-ODN didn't induce strong Th1 immune responses or inflammatory marker expression in 33 weeks.

In AD patients, skin lesions show a chronically relapsing inflammatory disorder with prurience and eczema. Therefore, we examined the effect of CpG-ODN on the appearance of skin lesions in CONV NC/Nga mice. In untreated-NC/Nga mice and non-CpG-ODN-treated mice, eczematous injuries were observed on the back, which resembles the typical features of AD. Compared to the control mice and non-CpG-ODN-treated mice, a drastic decrease in these injuries was observed in the CpG-ODN-treated mice. The number of these eczematous lesions was significantly decreased.

Histochemical examination of the lesions in CONV NC/Nga mice revealed hyperkeratosis, acanthosis, and parakeratosis, all of which are typical features of the skin of patients with AD. The infiltration of lymphocytes, macrophages, mast cells, and eosinophils was observed in the skin lesions. To analyze the effect of CpG-ODN on skin hypertrophy and granulocyte infiltration in CONV NC/Nga mice, CpG-ODN-treated skin was stained and examined with an optical microscope. An acanthosis was clearly suppressed in the CpG-ODN-treated mice compared with the control mice. Moreover, granulocyte and mast cell infiltration were decreased in the CpG-ODN-treated mice. These results indicate that CpG-ODN changes not only the Th2-predominant immune response in CONV NC/Nga mice but also the skin conditions, skin hypertrophy and mast cell infiltration.

To clarify the mechanisms of this effect of CpG-ODN, we first focused on the change in cytokine levels of the skin. Surprisingly, the mRNA levels of TGF-β and IL-10, cytokines which are considered to suppress inflammation especially in immune diseases, increased following transdermal application of CpG-ODN. Furthermore, we examined the mRNA expression of foxp-3, a marker of regulatory T cells (Tregs), because Tregs produce immune suppressive cytokines, TGF-β and IL-10. As expected, foxp-3 was expressed in the CpG-ODN-treated skin, which also expressed TGF-β and IL-10. These findings suggest that the up-regulations of TGF-β and IL-10 mRNA expression results in Treg being generated in the skin. Furthermore, $CD4^+CD25^+$ double-positive and $foxp3^+$ cells were observed only in the CpG-ODN-treated skin. These results indicate that CpG-ODN induces the induction and migration of Tregs in the skin of CONV NC/Nga mice.

In summary, CpG-ODN remarkably changed the immune response from type Th2 to Th1 as determined from cytokine mRNA and antibody levels. CpG-ODN induced Tregs to appear in the skin lesions. These results suggest that CpG-ODN could change cytokine production and generate Tregs in CONV NC/Nga mice, and may be effective for immunotherapy in patients with AD (Figure 4).

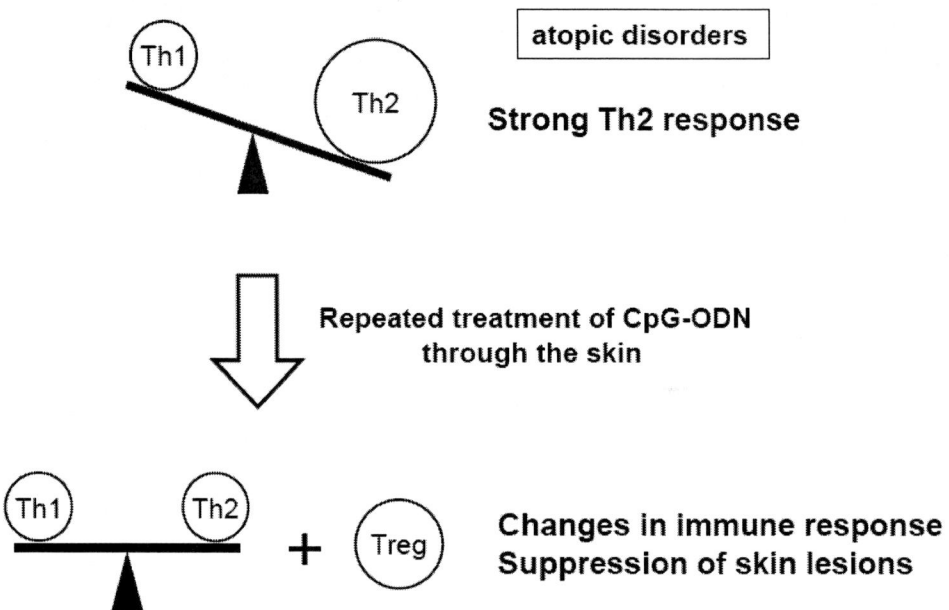

Figure 4. Changes in immune responses in NC/Nga mice.

Conclusion

Our findings suggested that transcutaneous vaccination with a COX-2 inhibitor induces efficient Th1 priming [32]. Th1-dominant immunity plays a critical role in the induction of anti-tumor immunity multiple helper functions, such as the capacity to enhance CTL priming of APCs, promote migration, proliferation, and cytotoxicity of tumor-specific CTLs. Additionally, the ability of CpG-ODN to shift the immune response from type Th2 to Th1 is expected to be used in immunotherapy for patients with diseases like AD that are associated with a Th2-predominant immune response. Our results showed that CpG-ODN remarkably changed the immune response from type Th2 to Th1 while inducing Tregs in skin lesions [54]. Thus, the skin is the one of the most promising sites for vaccination and immunotherapy for AD.

CpG-ODN induces strong a Th1-type immune response; however, CpG-ODN induces Tregs with a strong immune-suppressive function as well. Why does CpG-ODN have a directly-opposed function? One of the answers might be the dose of CpG-ODN. It has been reported that repeated or high doses of CpG-ODN induces strongly reduced immune responses [56-58]. In our case, a low dose of CpG-ODN was used for a tumor vaccine and a repeated high dose of CpG-ODN was used for AD. Additionally, COX-2 inhibitor suppresses PGE_2 and IL-10 productions that are the key cytokines for generation of Tregs by CpG-ODN. Furthermore, it was reported that the expression of COX-2 in Tregs controls their immune suppressive function [59]. Many other reasons take part in this phenomenon and more studies are needed for the explanation. All these results suggest that the regulation of immune response by CpG-ODNs is not simple, but it can be controlled with a dose of CpG-ODN and use COX-2 inhibitor together. In fact, our findings showed the administration of a COX-2 inhibitor with CpG-ODN through the skin enhances Th1-immune responses, but i.p. and i.v. had no effect.

In all senses, vaccination with CpG-ODN through the skin is a very simple and cost-effective strategy for tumor vaccines and immunotherapy in patients with AD and should be readily achievable.

References

[1] Seo, N., Tokura, Y., Nishijima, T., Hashizume, H., Furukawa, F. and Takigawa, M. (2000). Percutaneous peptide immunization via corneum barrier-disrupted murine skin for experimental tumor immunoprophylaxis. *Proc. Natl. Acad. Sci. U S A, 97,* 371-376.

[2] Takigawa, M., Tokura, Y., Hashizume, H., Yagi, H. and Seo, N. (2001). Percutaneous peptide immunization via corneum barrier-disrupted murine skin for experimental tumor immunoprophylaxis. *Ann. N Y Acad. Sci, 941,* 139-146.

[3] Bins, A.D., Jorritsma, A., Wolkers, M.C., Hung, C.F., Wu, T.C., Schumacher, T.N. and Haanen, J.B. (2005). A rapid and potent DNA vaccination strategy defined by in vivo monitoring of antigen expression. *Nat Med, 11,* 899-904.

[4] Kahlon, R., Hu, Y., Orteu, C.H., Kifayet, A., Trudeau, J.D., Tan, R. and Dutz, J.P. (2003). Optimization of epicutaneous immunization for the induction of CTL. *Vaccine, 21,* 2890-2899.

[5] Klimuk, S.K., Najar, H.M., Semple, S.C., Aslanian, S. and Dutz, J.P. (2004). Epicutaneous application of CpG oligodeoxynucleotides with peptide or protein antigen promotes the generation of CTL. *J Invest Dermatol, 122,* 1042-1049.

[6] Beignon, A.S., Briand, J.P., Muller, S. and Partidos, C.D. (2002). Immunization onto bare skin with synthetic peptides: immunomodulation with a CpG-containing oligodeoxynucleotide and effective priming of influenza virus-specific CD4[+] T cells. *Immunology, 105,* 204-212.

[7] Zhao, Y.L., Murthy, S.N., Manjili, M.H., Guan, L.J., Sen, A. and Hui, S.W. (2005). Induction of cytotoxic T-lymphocytes by electroporation-enhanced needle-free skin immunization. *Vaccine, 24,* 1282-1290.

[8] Kendall, M. (2006). Engineering of needle-free physical methods to target epidermal cells for DNA vaccination. *Vaccine, 24,* 4651-4656.

[9] Strid, J., Hourihane, J., Kimber, I., Callard, R. and Strobel, S. (2004). Disruption of the stratum corneum allows potent epicutaneous immunization with protein antigens resulting in a dominant systemic Th2 response. *Eur J Immunol, 34,* 2100-2109.

[10] Krieg, A.M. (2002). CpG motifs in bacterial DNA and their immune effects. *Annu Rev Immunol, 20,* 709-760.

[11] Agrawal, S. and Kandimalla, E.R. (2003). Modulation of Toll-like Receptor 9 Responses through Synthetic Immunostimulatory Motifs of DNA. *Ann N Y Acad Sci, 1002,* 30-42.

[12] Hemmi, H., Kaisho, T., Takeda, K. and Akira, S. (2003). The roles of Toll-like receptor 9, MyD88, and DNA-dependent protein kinase catalytic subunit in the effects of two distinct CpG DNAs on dendritic cell subsets. *J Immunol, 170,* 3059-3064.

[13] Spies, B., Hochrein, H., Vabulas, M., Huster, K., Busch, D.H., Schmitz, F., Heit, A. and Wagner, H. (2003). Vaccination with plasmid DNA activates dendritic cells via Toll-like receptor 9 (TLR9) but functions in TLR9-deficient mice. *J Immunol, 171,* 5908-5912.

[14] Davis, H.L., Weeratna, R., Waldschmidt, T.J., Tygrett, L., Schorr, J. and Krieg, A.M. (1998). CpG DNA is a potent enhancer of specific immunity in mice immunized with recombinant hepatitis B surface antigen. *J Immunol, 160,* 870-876

[15] Miconnet, I., Koenig, S., Speiser, D., Krieg, A., Guillaume, P., Cerottini, J.C. and Romero, P. (2002). CpG are efficient adjuvants for specific CTL induction against tumor antigen-derived peptide. *J Immunol, 168,* 1212-1218.

[16] Klinman, D.M., Currie, D., Gursel, I. and Verthelyi, D. (2004). Use of CpG oligodeoxynucleotides as immune adjuvants. *Immunol Rev, 199,* 201-216.

[17] Fiorentino, D.F., Bond, M.W. and Mosmann, T.R. (1989). Two types of mouse T helper cell. IV. Th2 clones secrete a factor that inhibits cytokine production by Th1 clones. *J Exp Med, 170,* 2081-2095.

[18] Mosmann, T.R. and Coffman, R.L. (1989). TH1 and TH2 cells: different patterns of lymphokine secretion lead to different functional properties. *Annu Rev Immunol, 7,* 145-173.

[19] Tuttle, T.M., McCrady, C.W., Inge, T.H., Salour, M. and Bear, H.D. (1993). gamma-Interferon plays a key role in T-cell-induced tumor regression. *Cancer Res, 53,* 833-839.

[20] Grewe, M., Bruijnzeel-Koomen, C.A., Schopf, E., Thepen, T., Langeveld-Wildschut, A.G., Ruzicka, T. and Krutmann, J. (1998). A role for Th1 and Th2 cells in the immunopathogenesis of atopic dermatitis. *Immunol. Today, 19,* 359-361.

[21] Spergel, J.M., Mizoguchi, E., Oettgen, H., Bhan, A. K. and Geha, R. S. (1999). Roles of TH1 and TH2 cytokines in a murine model of allergic dermatitis. *J. Clin. Invest, 103,* 1103-1111.

[22] Vestergaard, C., Yoneyama, H., Murai, M., Nakamura, K., Tamaki, K., Terashima, Y., Imai, T., Yoshie, O., Irimura, T., Mizutani, H., and Matsushima, K. (1999). Overproduction of Th2-specific chemokines in NC/Nga mice exhibiting atopic dermatitis-like lesions. *J. Clin. Invest, 104,* 1097-1105.

[23] van Bever, H. P. (1992). Recent advances in the pathogenesis of atopic dermatitis. *Eur. J. Pediatr, 151,* 870-873.

[24] Nakayama, H. (1996). Atopic dermatitis. *Dermatology, 38,* 484

[25] Escobar-Chávez, J.J., Merino-Sanjuán, V., López-Cervantes, M., Urban-Morlan, Z., Piñón-Segundo, E., Quintanar-Guerrero, D. and Ganem-Quintanar, A. (2008). The tape-stripping technique as a method for drug quantification in skin. *J Pharm Pharm Sci, 11,* 104-130.

[26] Moser, K., Kriwet, K., Naik, A., Kalia, Y.N. and Guy, R.H. (2001).Passive skin penetration enhancement and its quantification in vitro. *Eur J Pharmaceut Biopharm*, *52*, 103-112.

[27] Inoue, J., Yotsumoto, S., Sakamoto, T., Tsuchiya, S. and Aramaki, Y. (2005). Changes in immune responses to antigen applied to tape-stripped skin with CpG-oligodeoxynucleotide in mice. *J. Control. Release, 108*, 294-305.

[28] Inoue, J., Yotsumoto, S., Sakamoto, T., Tsuchiya, S. and Aramaki, Y. (2005). Changes in immune responses to antigen applied to tape-stripped skin with CpG-oligodeoxynucleotide in NC/Nga mice. *Pharm. Res, 22,* 1627-1633.

[29] I Inoue, J., Yotsumoto, S., Sakamoto, T., Tsuchiya, S. and Aramaki, Y. (2006). Changes in immune responses to mite antigen sensitized through barrier-disrupted skin with CpG-oligodeoxynucleotide in mice. *Biol Pharm Bull, 29,* 385-387.

[30] Inoue, J. and Aramaki, Y. (2007). Toll-like receptor-9 expression induced by tape-stripping triggers on effective immune response with CpG-oligodeoxynucleotides. *Vaccine, 25,* 1007-1013.

[31] Glenn, G.M., Kenney, R.T., Ellingsworth, L.R., Frech, S.A., Hammond, S.A. and Zoeteweij, J.P. (2003). Transcutaneous immunization and immunostimulant strategies: capitalizing on the immunocompetence of the skin. *Expert Rev Vaccines, 2,* 253-267.

[32] Inoue, J. and Aramaki, Y. (2007). Cyclooxygenase-2 inhibition promotes enhancement of antitumor responses by transcutaneous vaccination with cytosine-phosphate-guanosine-oligodeoxynucleotides and model tumor antigen. *J Invest Dermatol, 127,* 614-621

[33] Howe, L.R., Chang, S.H., Tolle, K.C., Dillon, R., Young, L.J., Cardiff, R.D., Newman, R.A., Yang, P., Thaler, H.T., Muller, W.J., Hudis, C., Brown, A.M., Hla, T., Subbaramaiah, K. and Dannenberg, A.J. (2005). HER2/neu-induced mammary tumorigenesis and angiogenesis are reduced in cyclooxygenase-2 knockout mice. *Cancer Res, 65,* 10113-10119.

[34] Sharma, S., Yang, S.C., Zhu, L., Reckamp, K., Gardner, B., Baratelli, F., Huang, M., Batra, R.K. and Dubinett, S.M. (2005). Tumor cyclooxygenase-2/prostaglandin E2-dependent promotion of FOXP3 expression and CD4+ CD25+ T regulatory cell activities in lung cancer. *Cancer Res, 65,* 5211-5220.

[35] Chen, Y., Zhang, J., Moore, S.A., Ballas, Z.K., Portanova, J.P., Krieg, A.M. and Berg, D.J. (2001). CpG DNA induces cyclooxygenase-2 expression and prostaglandin production. *Int Immunol, 13,* 1013-1020.

[36] Ghosh, D.K., Misukonis, M.A., Reich, C., Pisetsky, D.S. and Weinberg, J.B. (2001). Host response to infection: the role of CpG DNA in induction of cyclooxygenase 2 and nitric oxide synthase 2 in murine macrophages. *Infect Immun, 69,* 7703-7710.

[37] Katamura, K., Shintaku, N., Yamauchi, Y., Fukui, T., Ohshima, Y., Mayumi, M. and Furusho, K. (1995). Prostaglandin E2 at priming of naive $CD4^+$ T cells inhibits acquisition of ability to produce IFN-gamma and IL-2, but not IL-4 and IL-5. *J Immunol, 155,* 4604-4612.

[38] Abe, N., Katamura, K., Shintaku, N., Fukui, T., Kiyomasu, T., Iio, J., Ueno, H., Tai, G., Mayumi, M. and Furusho, K. (1997). Prostaglandin E2 and IL-4 provide naive $CD4^+$ T

cells with distinct inhibitory signals for the priming of IFN-gamma production. *Cell Immunol, 181,* 86-89.

[39] Wu, C.Y., Wang, K., McDyer, J.F. and Seder, R.A. (1998). Prostaglandin E2 and dexamethasone inhibit IL-12 receptor expression and IL-12 responsiveness. *J Immunol, 161,* 2723-2730.

[40] Harizi, H., Juzan, M., Pitard, V., Moreau, J.F. and Gualde, N. (2002). Cyclooxygenase-2-issued prostaglandin e(2) enhances the production of endogenous IL-10, which down-regulates dendritic cell functions. *J Immunol, 168,* 2255-2263.

[41] Yi, A.K., Yoon, J.G., Yeo, S.J., Hong, S.C., English, B.K. and Krieg, A.M. (2002). Role of mitogen-activated protein kinases in CpG DNA-mediated IL-10 and IL-12 production: central role of extracellular signal-regulated kinase in the negative feedback loop of the CpG DNA-mediated Th1 response. *J Immunol, 168,* 4711-4720.

[42] Wang, B., Zhuang, L., Fujisawa, H., Shinder, G.A., Feliciani, C., Shivji, G.M., Suzuki, H., Amerio, P., Toto, P., Sauder, D.N. (1999). Enhanced epidermal Langerhans cell migration in IL-10 knockout mice. *J Immunol, 162,* 277-283.

[43] Hsieh, C.S., Macatonia, S.E., Tripp, C.S., Wolf, S.F., O'Garra, A. and Murphy, K.M. (1993). Development of TH1 CD4[+] T cells through IL-12 produced by Listeria-induced macrophages. *Science, 260,* 547-549.

[44] Trinchieri, G. (1993). Interleukin-12 and its role in the generation of TH1 cells. *Immunol Today, 14,* 335-338.

[45] Nakamura, H.., Aoki, M., Tamai, K., Oishi, M., Ogihara, T., Kaneda, Y. and Morishita, R. (2002). Prevention and regression of atopic dermatitis by ointment containing NF-kB decoy oligodeoxynucleotides in NC/Nga atopic mouse model. *Gene. Ther, 9,* 1221-1229.

[46] Leung, D.Y., Boguniewicz, M., Howell, M.D., Nomura, I. and Hamid. Q.A. (2004). New insights into atopic dermatitis. *J. Clin. Invest, 113,* 651-657.

[47] Cooper, K.D. (1994). Atopic dermatitis: recent trends in pathogenesis and therapy. *J. Invest. Dermatol, 102,* 128-137.

[48] Rudikoff, D. and Lebwohl, M. (1998). Atopic dermatitis. *Lancet, 351,* 1715-1721.

[49] Soter, N.A. (1989). Morphology of atopic eczema. *Allergy, 44,* 16-19.

[50] Uehara, M., Izukura, R. and Sawai, T. (1990). Blood eosinophilia in atopic dermatitis. *Clin. Exp. Dermatol, 15,* 264-266.

[51] Kondo, K., Nagami, T. and Todokoro, S. (1969). Differences in haematopoietic death among inbred strains of mice. *Tokyo. Igakusyoin,* 20.

[52] Vestergaard, C., Yoneyama, H. and Matsushima, K. (2000). The NC/Nga mouse: a model for atopic dermatitis. *Mol. Med. Today, 6,* 209-210.

[53] Matsuda, H., Watanabe, N., Geba, G.P., Sperl, J., Tsudzuki, M., Hiroi, J., Matsumoto, M., Ushio, H., Saito, S., Askenase, P.W. and Ra, C. (1997). Development of atopic dermatitis-like skin lesion with IgE hyperproduction in NC/Nga mice. *Int. Immunol, 9,* 461-466.

[54] Inoue, J. and Aramaki, Y. (2007). Suppression of skin lesions by transdermal application of CpG-oligodeoxynucleotides in NC/Nga mice, a model of human atopic dermatitis. *J Immunol, 178,* 584-591.

[55] Imokawa, G., Abe, A., Jin, K., Higaki, Y., Kawashima, M. and Hidano, A. (1991). Decreased level of ceramides in stratum corneum of atopic dermatitis: an etiologic factor in atopic dry skin? *J. Invest. Dermatol, 96,* 523-526.

[56] Mellor, A.L., Baban, B., Chandler, P.R., Manlapat, A., Kahler, D.J. and Munn, D.H. (2005). CpG oligonucleotides induce splenic CD19+ dendritic cells to acquire potent indoleamine 2,3-dioxygenase-dependent T cell regulatory functions via IFN Type 1 signaling. *J Immunol, 175,* 5601-5605.

[57] Wingender, G., Garbi, N., Schumak, B., Jüngerkes, F., Endl, E., von Bubnoff, D., Steitz, J., Striegler, J., Moldenhauer, G., Tüting, T., Heit, A., Huster, K.M., Takikawa, O., Akira, S., Busch, D.H., Wagner, H., Hämmerling, G.J., Knolle, P.A. and Limmer, A. (2006). Systemic application of CpG-rich DNA suppresses adaptive T cell immunity via induction of IDO. *Eur J Immunol, 36,* 12-20.

[58] Hayashi, T., Beck, L., Rossetto, C., Gong, X., Takikawa, O., Takabayashi, K., Broide, D.H., Carson, D.A. and Raz, E. (2004). Inhibition of experimental asthma by indoleamine 2,3-dioxygenase. *J Clin Invest, 114,* 270-279.

[59] Mahic, M., Yaqub, S., Johansson, C.C., Taskén, K. and Aandahl, E.M. (2006). FOXP3+CD4+CD25+ adaptive regulatory T cells express cyclooxygenase-2 and suppress effector T cells by a prostaglandin E2-dependent mechanism. *J. Immunol, 177,* 246-254.

Reviewed by Prof. Naohito Ohno[*].
*Laboratory for Immunopharmacology of Microbial Products, School of Pharmacy, Tokyo University of Pharmacy and Life Sciences

In: Immunologic Adjuvant Research
Editor: Antonio H. Benvenuto

ISBN 978-1-60692-399-3
© 2009 Nova Science Publishers, Inc.

Chapter 4

Immunopotentiating Reconstituted Influenza Virosomes as Safe and Potent Antigen-Delivery System for Synthetic Peptides in Vaccine Development

Claudia A. Daubenberger [3]*1, Gerd Pluschke* [1]*, Rinaldo Zurbriggen* [2]*, and Nicole Westerfeld* [2]

1 Swiss Tropical Institute, Molecular Immunology, 4002 Basel, Switzerland
2 Pevion Biotech, Worblentalstrasse 32, CH - 3063 Bern

Abstract

The development of effective vaccines for malaria, tuberculosis and HIV represents one of the most important scientific public health challenges of our time. One possible approach is based on subunit vaccines that utilize well defined antigens for which there is evidence of protective immunity from epidemiological data in the field or animal challenge models. In malaria vaccine development, it is generally accepted that an effective subunit vaccine will target antigens of several developmental stages of the parasite *Plasmodium falciparum*. Currently, the development of subunit vaccines is hampered by their poor immunogenicity and lack of suitable antigen delivery systems driving appropriate immune responses in humans. Most importantly, the recombinant proteins or synthetic peptides delivered have to mimic closely the corresponding native malaria protein to induce effective antibody responses. Here we focus on novel concepts in malaria vaccine development highlighting recent advances in the design of synthetic vaccine candidates and antigen delivery systems based on immuno-potentiating reconstituted influenza virosomes.

---

[3] Corresponding author: Claudia A. Daubenberger, Swiss Tropical Institute, Socinstrasse 57, 4002 Basel, Switzerland, phone: +41 61 2848217; fax: +41 61 2718654, e-mail: Claudia.Daubenberger@unibas.ch.

Vaccines are likely to represent the most cost-effective public health interventions available. The problem of emerging and re-emerging infectious diseases underscores the need for more effective vaccine technologies in future [1]. Live vaccines have intrinsic immunogenic properties that make them ideal immunogens inducing long-lived immunity with efficient and appropriate B and T cell responses. However, not all pathogens can be attenuated to be used as live vaccines particularly due to serious safety concerns in immuno-compromised subjects within a given population [2].

Subunit vaccines based on recombinant proteins or synthetic peptides are not confronted with these concerns but their increased safety is accompanied with lower immunogenicity. To promote protective immune responses, the addition of adjuvants is required for activation of appropriate arms of the adaptive immune system. Although no examples of commercially available synthetic peptide based vaccines currently exist, this type of vaccine has intrinsic advantages that will be harnessed in future. Using this approach, humoral immune responses can be focussed to generate a preferred repertoire of antibodies that target defined epitopes known for their ability to afford protection. Induction of unprotective humoral immunity often shown or at least suspected to be involved in immune evasion mechanisms can thus be avoided [3]. For successful vaccination, antibodies which recognize the cognate, native antigen (cross-reactive immunogenicity) and neutralize the infectivity of the pathogen (cross-protective immunogenicity) expressing this antigen have to be elicited. When combined with an appropriate adjuvant most peptides are immunogenic, i.e. they readily induce antibodies that react with the peptide immunogen itself. Analysis of three dimensional structures of antibody – peptide complexes has however shown that the majority of epitopes are discontinuous which explains why most antibodies raised against a native protein will not cross-react with short linear peptide fragments delineated from this molecule. Since it has been challenging to artificially reconstitute discontinuous B cell epitopes by chemical synthesis for use as immunogens [4], efforts have been mainly focused on the use of linear peptides representing continuous epitopes. Linear peptides are easy to synthesize but suffer from serious drawbacks including limited bio-availability due to rapid degradation in biological fluids and the fact that the B cell receptor repertoire encounters a range of accessible conformational states available to the peptide that is not necessarily mimicking the native structure of the protein targeted [5]. In fact, for most continuous epitopes of viruses described in the literature, there is no evidence that they initiate the required cross-reactive and cross-protective humoral immune responses [6]. A further difficulty arises from the intrinsically weak immunogenicity of peptides shorter than 40 amino acids, which usually necessitates conjugation to carrier molecules. When several peptide moieties are coupled to a protein carrier, the microenvironment at each point of peptide attachment is likely to be different leading to altered conformations of the peptide [7;8]. Additionally, the carrier itself can induce ineffective bystander immune responses, possibly interfering negatively with the initiation of desired immune responses. Several of these issues have been addressed successfully by us using conformationally constrained synthetic peptides selected in iterative identification procedures to finally arrive at native-like peptide conformations delivered on the surface of immuno-potentiating reconstituted influenza virosomes (IRIV).

Mechanisms underlying the excellent immunogenicity of viruses have been elucidated in the recent years. These include the highly repetitive and ordered surface structures, their particulate nature and ability to induce innate immunity via pathogen associated molecular patterns interacting with pattern recognition receptors for appropriate conditioning of host adaptive immune responses [9] These features can serve as paradigm for rational vaccine design and many new generation vaccines are trying to make use of these properties [10].

Almeida et al., developed the first IRIV from influenza virus in 1975 [11]. Hemaglutinin (HA) and neuraminidase (NA) removed from the influenza virus envelope were purified and reassembled on the surface of unilamellar liposomes. These structures resembled the original virus with a mean diameter of 100-200 nm and spike-like components of 10 – 15 nm similar to influenza HA. Essentially, IRIV can be regarded as liposomes carrying on their surface the two glycoproteins HA and NA lacking infectious RNA. Major constituents of IRIV are 70 % phosphatidylcholine, 20 % phosphatidylethanolamine and 10 % envelope phospholipids from H1N1 influenza virus A/Singapore strain. IRIV can be used for vaccine development, drug delivery, or gene transfer [12]. The NA is a tetramer composed of four equal, spherical subunits hydrophobically embedded in the IRIV membrane by a central stalk. HA, the major influenza antigen, is formed by two polypeptides, HA1 and HA2. Surface exposed HA stabilizes the liposome structure by prevention of fusion with other liposomes. Influenza infection starts with the binding of the HA to N-acetylneuraminic acid components of various host cell surface glycoproteins or glycolipids including the surface of antigen presenting cells such as macrophages. It is thought that HA therefore facilitates the binding of IRIV to these cells that are important for the activation of both the innate and adaptive immune system, channelling bound antigens directly to antigen processing and presentation pathways. The fusion of IRIV with endosomal membranes is mediated by the HA2 polypeptide enabling the targeting of proteins into the MHC class I or class II pathway, depending on how the antigens are presented to the antigen presenting cells. Antigens linked to the surface of IRIV are presented to the immune system in a highly repetitive mode activating B cells by cross-linking surface Ig specific for these structures. In parallel, the antigens are degraded upon fusion within the endosomes and then presented in the context of MHC class II molecules potentially stimulating CD4 helper T cells. Antigens that have been encapsulated within the virosome are delivered to the cytosol, thus entering the MHC class I pathway and stimulating CD8 T cells. Because of their intrinsic adjuvant activity due to induction of cytokines like GM-CSF, TNF-α, INF-γ and IL-2 in peripheral blood mononuclear cells (PBMC) and the antigen depot effect, IRIV enhance immunogenicity of coupled structures delivered in conjunction with the virosomes [13]. Two vaccines based on IRIV are licensed for human use, namely Epaxal® and Inflexal®. These are vaccines preventing the viral diseases hepatitis A and influenza, most likely through the efficient triggering of a humoral response. These formulations have an excellent safety/efficiency profile demonstrated by > 45 mio doses applied to date [14].

When using IRIV as adjuvant and carrier system for synthetic peptides, it is essential to physically associate the antigen of interest with the virosomal particle to employ the full adjuvant activity [15]. The delivered peptide may either be associated with the surface or encapsulated within the virosomal particle. For surface exposure, the N or C-terminus of the peptide is coupled to phosphatidylethanolamine (PE) via chemical cross-linking. The resulting peptide-PE conjugate is integrated into the membrane via the lipid moiety and exposes the peptide structure on the surface of the IRIV. Important for the superior activity of influenza virosomes as antigen delivery system compared to liposomes is a strong pre-existing immunity to the carrier itself [16]. The importance of pre-existing influenza immune memory has been demonstrated by comparing the potency of peptide-bearing virosomes in mice with and without pre-immunisation against influenza [16;17]. Clearly, presence of influenza virus memory improved considerably the antibody responses specific for the delivered synthetic peptide while it did not influence the immunogenicity of peptide antigens encapsulated in the particle to elicit cytotoxic T cell responses [18]. The mechanisms behind might be represented by the expanded number of memory T cells recognizing HA that provide help to B cells recognizing the surface bound synthetic peptide. Additionally, presence of antibodies binding to virosomes could enhance the uptake of the particles by antigen-presenting cells via opsonization [14]. When considering vaccines for countries in sub-Saharan Africa, temperature sensitivity is a critical parameter. Continuous cold-chains may not be available during transport in these countries, thus, vaccines need to maintain their function even upon prolonged exposure to elevated temperatures. This is achieved now by a new generation of stabilized virosomes (TIRIV) that can be lyophilized without loss of either fusogenic or immuno-potentiating properties by modifications of the formulation method and inclusion of certain molecules (="T") stabilizing the particle structure during the lyophilization process [19].

The aim of a multi-stage multi-valent subunit malaria vaccine is to focus immune responses onto protection-mediating structural elements of parasite proteins. It is generally accepted that anti-peptide antibodies cross-reacting with the parent protein will be obtained if the conformation of the peptide immunogen resembles closely the corresponding segment of the parent protein. Producing synthetic peptides that mirror closely the malaria protein is therefore one of the cornerstones of peptide based vaccine development approach. *P. falciparum* candidate proteins were chosen on the basis of known essential function in the host cell invasion. Criteria for peptide selection included i) target of parasite growth inhibitory antibodies, ii) proposed essential role in parasite development, iii) amino acid sequence conservation and iv) secondary structure motifs indicating surface exposition. Based on these criteria, the design of conformationally constrained synthetic peptides was optimized using sequential rounds of structure optimization as applied in drug development. The key read out was the parasite-binding properties of antibodies elicited in mice after immunisation with the corresponding peptide coupled to the surface of IRIV. The circumsporozoite protein (CSP), the major surface protein of the incoming sporozoite, has been the focus of numerous efforts over many years to develop a pre-erythrocytic vaccine preventing hepatocyte invasion [20]. The CSP forms a dense coat covering the entire surface of the sporozoite and it has been shown that CSP is critical for sporozoite localization and development of the liver stage of the parasite [21;22]. CSP from all species of *Plasmodium* have a similar overall structure composed of a central species-specific repeat region, a highly conserved cell-adhesive sequence in the carboxy-terminus of the protein with similarity to the type I thrombospondin repeat and a highly conserved 5 amino acid sequence called region I, just upstream of the repeats [20]. Antibodies against CSP are primarily directed against the central repeat region, with minor B cell epitopes mapped to non-repeat flanking regions. The existence of a safe and reliable human challenge model that incorporates a standardized sporozoite challenge has revealed that the most promising CSP-derived experimental vaccine candidates include immuno-dominant B cell epitopes present in the central NANP region and T cell epitopes from the C terminal portion of the molecule [23]. Nuclear magnetic resonance (NMR) spectroscopy studies on linear peptides containing one or several tandemly linked NANP motifs suggested the presence of turn-like structures based on the NANP cadence, stabilized by hydrogen bonding remaining in rapid dynamic equilibrium with extended chain forms [24]. A crystal structure has been reported of the pentapeptide Ac-ANPNA-NH$_2$ which confirmed that the NANP motif adopts a type-I β-turn conformation stabilized by hydrogen bonding [25]. A conformationally defined synthetic peptide based on the NANP-repeat region of CSP has been developed by us building on NMR and modelling studies [17;26-28]. This synthetic peptide has been named UK-39 and represents a circularized structure of five NANP repeats. Immunisation of mice and rabbits with UK-39 coupled to the surface of IRIV resulted in high titres of sporozoite cross-reactive antibodies. UK-39 was recognized by all tested CSP-repeat region specific monoclonal antibodies elicited by sporozoite immunization of mice and by the majority of sera from human donors living in malaria endemic regions [26]. UK-39 specific monoclonal antibodies and IgG purified from sera of UK-39 immunized rabbits and humans inhibited the invasion of hepatocytes by *P. falciparum* sporozoites providing evidence for protective capacity [26].

The apical membrane antigen-1 (AMA-1), a leading malaria asexual blood stage vaccine candidate has been selected as second candidate antigen [29]. AMA-1 is required for sporozoite invasion of hepatocytes [30] and merozoite invasion of erythrocytes [31]. AMA-1 is targeted to the micronemes of developing merozoites and is initially expressed as an 83 kDa precursor protein [32]. N-terminal processing produces a 66 kDa product that is released onto the surface of the free merozoite [33]. At the time of invasion, AMA-1 is cleaved by a membrane-bound subtilisin-like protease, PfSUB2, resulting in the shedding of a 48 kDa fragment and only the cytoplasmic, trans-membrane, and a 29 residue membrane-adjacent fragment can be detected in ring-stage parasites [34]. Vaccination with recombinant AMA-1 induces protection against homologous parasite challenge in both rodents and monkeys [35;36] and antibodies to AMA-1 have been shown to inhibit erythrocyte invasion and parasite growth *in vitro* [37]. A cyclized synthetic peptide (AMA49-C1) of 49 amino acids comprising residues 446 to 490 of AMA-1 (semi-conserved loop I of domain III) has been shown to induce parasite-growth inhibitory antibodies in mice after delivery as surface bound peptide by IRIV [38].

After pre-clinical development, safety and immunogenicity of IRIV-based formulations of the two selected and optimized peptide structures was tested in a phase Ia clinical trial in Basel, Switzerland [39]. Five groups of eight subjects received virosomal formulations containing 10 μg or 50 μg of AMA49-C1, the AMA-1 derived synthetic phosphatidyl-ethanolamine (PE-)-peptide conjugate [38] or 10 μg or 50 μg of UK-39, the CSP derived synthetic PE-peptide conjugate [26] or 50 μg of both antigens each. A control group of six subjects received mock virosomes. Virosomal formulations of the peptides AMA49-C1 (designated PEV301) and UK-39 (designated PEV302) were injected i.m. on days 0, 60 and 180. No serious or severe adverse events related to the vaccine were observed and both PEV301 and PEV302 elicited already after two injections a synthetic peptide-specific antibody response assessed by ELISA in all volunteers immunized with the appropriate antigen dose [39]. The impact of UK-39 specific antibodies on sporozoite infectivity, sporozoite migration through hepatocytes (HepG2 cell line) and sporozoite invasion of human primary hepatocyte cultures was assessed using purified IgG from immunized volunteers. Vaccination induced migration inhibitory activity was observed in seven out of seven subjects immunized with PEV302 and sporozoite invasion inhibition was observed in six out of the seven volunteers. IgG preparations from controls immunized with PEV301 or IRIV alone did not interfere with sporozoite migration or invasion. Antibody titres assessed in ELISA correlated closely with *in vitro* inhibition of sporozoite migration and invasion of hepatocytes [40]. Invasion inhibition correlated positively with migration inhibition, suggesting that anti-UK-39 antibodies interfered with parasite gliding motility, which is based on the same mechanism of redistribution of proteins along the sporozoite surface as host cell invasion [41]. These results confirmed that the UK-39 peptido-mimetic closely resembles the natural conformation of the NANP repeats expressed on the sporozoite surface [40]. Increases in anti-UK-39 antibody avidity over the course of immunisations indicated that B cell memory has been induced. The combined delivery of two different synthetic peptides did not interfere with the immunogenicity of single components [40]. One year after the third immunisation 10 out of 11 volunteers were still positive for parasite-binding antibodies indicating that the immune responses are long-lived. Antibodies cross-reactive with UK-39 in ELISA and with CSP in Western blot analysis were detectable in the pre-immune serum of one volunteer. After vaccination, this pre-existing humoral immunity unrelated to a known history of malaria exposure was boosted exceptionally already by the first immunisation with UK-39, yielding the highest titres observed in the entire trial [40]. This observation might suggest that IRIV-based vaccines have the potential to boost natural malaria immunity.

The cellular immune responses specific for IRIV and the surface bound synthetic malaria peptides has been analysed. After vaccination, in 50 % (8/16) of the volunteers at least one positive lymphoproliferative response specific for the 49mer peptide derived from AMA-1 was observed with stimulation indices ranging from 2 to 4.5. As expected, no proliferative responses specific for UK-39 lacking HLA class II binding motifs was measured. All volunteers showed pre-existing IRIV specific cellular immunity assessed by *ex vivo* IFN-g ELISpot analysis and lympho-proliferation. Importantly, the strong pre-existing influenza specific T cell responses did not interfere negatively with the induction of malaria peptide specific humoral and cellular immune responses [19]. In a phase IIa clinical trial conducted at the Centre for Clinical Vaccinology and Tropical Medicine, University of Oxford, UK protection of immunized volunteers against sporozoite challenge was assessed [42]. This trial verified the safety and immunogenicity results of the phase Ia trial in Basel. Although the sporozoite challenge did not demonstrate sterile protection from liver infection, there were clear indications that the vaccine induced responses influencing the development of the parasites. The growth rate of asexual blood stage parasites was significantly lower in vaccinees compared to unvaccinated volunteers and four persons were able to partially control blood stage development of the parasite. One of these volunteer did not develop blood stage parasitemia until day 20, a delay that has never been observed in any unvaccinated volunteer. The immunization protocol led to changes of the parasite morphology of asexual blood stages (crisis form) in 100 % of the immunized persons [42]. Currently, a phase Ib trial in Tanzania with PEV301 and PEV302 is conducted to compare safety and immunogenicity results between malaria naïve European volunteers and malaria exposed and semi-immune people. The questions that will be addressed are whether natural immune responses against CSP and AMA-1 can be boosted by vaccination and to assess the influence of circulating malaria parasites on vaccine induced immune responses.

One outstanding advantage of the IRIV system compared to other malaria vaccine approaches is the principle of single building blocks, which can be combined into a multi-component subunit vaccine. Each building block, i.e. peptide derived from a *P. falciparum* antigen presented on the virosome surface can be produced and evaluated separately. Depending on the clinical trial results, distinct building blocks can be combined and delivered together in a single inoculation. Hence, a continuous vaccine optimisation process can be followed. So far, various peptides derived from different malaria antigens have been evaluated pre-clinically as additional components of the virosomal malaria vaccine. These include blood stage antigens like Merozoite Surface Protein 1 (MSP-1), MSP-3 and Serine Repeat Antigen 5. Peptides derived from these antigens have been tested and optimized to induce parasite interacting antibodies similar to the optimization process applied for AMA-1 and CSP derived peptides [43;44].

In summary, results of pre-clinical and clinical profiling showed that IRIV represent an vaccine antigen delivery platform that i) is safe and well-tolerated in humans, ii) can deliver multiple antigens from different developmental stages of *P. falciparum*, iii) induces peptide specific, parasite binding, affinity matured humoral immune responses after two inoculations in 100 % of vaccinees, iv) provokes durable humoral immune responses with antibodies detectable one year after last immunization, v) mounted humoral and cellular immune responses are not negatively influenced by pre-existing influenza immunity, vi) in which formulations can be quickly modified allowing agile responses to new synthetic peptide developments and vii) is safe for the environment.

References

[1] Almond JW. Vaccine renaissance. *Nat. Rev. Micro.* 2007; 5: 478-481.
[2] Plotkin SA. Vaccines, vaccination, and vaccinology. *J. Infect Dis.* 2003; 187: 1349-1359.
[3] Guevara Patino JA, Holder AA, McBride JS, Blackman MJ. Antibodies that Inhibit Malaria Merozoite Surface Protein-1 Processing and Erythrocyte Invasion Are Blocked by Naturally Acquired Human Antibodies. *J. Exp. Med.* 1997; 186: 1689-1699.
[4] Enshell-Seijffers D, Denisov D, Groisman B, Smelyanski L, Meyuhas R, Gross G, Denisova G, Gershoni JM. The Mapping and Reconstitution of a Conformational Discontinuous B-cell Epitope of HIV-1. *Journal of Molecular Biology* 2003; 334: 87-101.
[5] Bastian M, Lozano JM, Patarroyo ME, Pluschke G, Daubenberger CA. Characterization of a reduced peptide bond analogue of a promiscuous CD4 T cell epitope derived from the *Plasmodium falciparum* malaria vaccine candidate merozoite surface protein 1. *Mol. Immunol.* 2004; 41: 775-784.

[6] Van Regenmortel MH. The rational design of biological complexity: a deceptive metaphor. *Proteomics*. 2007; 7: 965-975.

[7] Friede M, Muller S, Briand JP, Plaue S, Fernandes I, Frisch B, Schuber F, Van Regenmortel MHV. Selective induction of protection against influenza virus infection in mice by a lipid-peptide conjugate delivered in liposomes. *Vaccine* 1994; 12: 791-797.

[8] Karle S, Nishiyama Y, Taguchi H, Zhou YX, Luo J, Planque S, Hanson C, Paul S. Carrier-dependent specificity of antibodies to a conserved peptide determinant of gp120. *Vaccine* 2003; 21: 1213-1218.

[9] Fehr T, Bachmann MF, Bucher E, Kalinke U, Di Padova FE, Lang AB, Hengartner H, Zinkernagel RM. Role of repetitive antigen patterns for induction of antibodies against antibodies. *J. Exp. Med.* 1997; 185: 1785-1792.

[10] Jennings GT, Bachmann MF. Designing recombinant vaccines with viral properties: a rational approach to more effective vaccines. *Curr. Mol. Med.* 2007; 7: 143-155.

[11] Almeida JD, Edwards DC, Brand CM, Heath TD. Formation of virosomes from influenza subunits and liposomes. *Lancet* 1975; 2: 899-901.

[12] Moser C, Amacker M, Kammer AR, Rasi S, Westerfeld N, Zurbriggen R. Influenza virosomes as a combined vaccine carrier and adjuvant system for prophylactic and therapeutic immunizations. *Expert Review of Vaccines* 2007; 6: 711-721.

[13] Schumacher R, Adamina M, Zurbriggen R, Bolli M, Padovan E, Zajac P, Heberer M, Spagnoli GC. Influenza virosomes enhance class I restricted CTL induction through CD4+ T cell activation. *Vaccine* 2004; 22: 714-723.

[14] Westerfeld N, Zurbriggen R. Peptides delivered by immunostimulating reconstituted influenza virosomes. *J. Pept. Sci.* 2005; 11: 707-712.

[15] Zurbriggen R, Novak-Hofer I, Seelig A, Gluck R. IRIV-adjuvanted hepatitis A vaccine: in vivo absorption and biophysical characterization. Prog. Lipid Res 2000; 39: 3-18.

[16] Zurbriggen R, Gluck R. Immunogenicity of. *Vaccine* 1999; 17: 1301-1305.

[17] Poltl-Frank F, Zurbriggen R, Helg A, Stuart F, Robinson J, Gluck R, Pluschke G. Use of reconstituted influenza virus virosomes as an immunopotentiating delivery system for a peptide-based vaccine. *Clin. Exp. Immunol.* 1999; 117: 496-503.

[18] Amacker M, Engler O, Kammer AR, Vadrucci S, Oberholzer D, Cerny A, Zurbriggen R. Peptide-loaded chimeric influenza virosomes for efficient in vivo induction of cytotoxic T cells. *Int. Immunol.* 2005; 17: 695-704.

[19] Peduzzi E, Westerfeld N, Zurbriggen R, Pluschke G, Daubenberger CA. Contribution of influenza immunity and virosomal-formulated synthetic peptide to cellular immune responses in a phase I subunit malaria vaccine trial. *Clin. Immunol.* 2008.

[20] Kappe SHI, Buscaglia CA, Nussenzweig V. Plasmodium Sporozoite Molecular Cell Biology. *Annual Review of Cell and Developmental Biology* 2004; 20: 29-59.

[21] Coppi A, Tewari R, Bishop JR, Bennett BL, Lawrence R, Esko JD, Billker O, Sinnis P. Heparan sulfate proteoglycans provide a signal to Plasmodium sporozoites to stop migrating and productively invade host cells. Cell Host. *Microbe* 2007; 2: 316-327.

[22] Singh AP, Buscaglia CA, Wang Q, Levay A, Nussenzweig DR, Walker JR, Winzeler EA, Fujii H, Fontoura BM, Nussenzweig V. Plasmodium circumsporozoite protein promotes the development of the liver stages of the parasite. *Cell* 2007; 131: 492-504.

[23] Stoute JA, Slaoui M, Heppner DG, Momin P, Kester KE, Desmons P, Wellde BT, Garcon N, Krzych U, Marchand M. A preliminary evaluation of a recombinant circumsporozoite protein vaccine against *Plasmodium falciparum* malaria. RTS,S Malaria Vaccine Evaluation Group. *N. Engl. J. Med* 1997; 336: 86-91.

[24] Dyson HJ, Satterthwait AC, Lerner RA, Wright PE. Conformational preferences of synthetic peptides derived from the immunodominant site of the circumsporozoite protein of *Plasmodium falciparum* by 1H NMR. *Biochemistry* 1990; 29: 7828-7837.

[25] Ghasparian A, Moehle K, Linden A, Robinson JA. Crystal structure of an NPNA-repeat motif from the circumsporozoite protein of the malaria parasite *Plasmodium falciparum*. Chemical Communications 174-176.

[26] Okitsu SL, Kienzl U, Moehle K, Silvie O, Peduzzi E, Mueller MS, Sauerwein RW, Matile H, Zurbriggen R, Mazier D, Robinson JA, Pluschke G. Structure-activity-based design of a synthetic malaria peptide eliciting sporozoite inhibitory antibodies in a virosomal formulation. *Chem. Biol.* 2007; 14: 577-587.

[27] Pfeiffer B, Peduzzi E, Moehle K, Zurbriggen R, Gluck R, Pluschke G, Robinson JA. A virosome-mimotope approach to synthetic vaccine design and optimization: synthesis, conformation, and immune recognition of a potential malaria-vaccine candidate. *Angew. Chem. Int. Ed. Engl.* 2003; 42: 2368-2371.

[28] Moreno R, Jiang L, Moehle K, Zurbriggen R, Gluck R, Robinson JA, Pluschke G. Exploiting conformationally constrained peptidomimetics and an efficient human-compatible delivery system in synthetic vaccine design. *Chembiochem.* 2001; 2: 838-843.

[29] Girard MP, Reed ZH, Friede M, Kieny MP. A review of human vaccine research and development: malaria. *Vaccine* 2007; 25: 1567-1580.

[30] Silvie O, Franetich JF, Charrin S, Mueller MS, Siau A, Bodescot M, Rubinstein E, Hannoun L, Charoenvit Y, Kocken CH, Thomas AW, van Gemert GJ, Sauerwein RW, Blackman MJ, Anders RF, Pluschke G, Mazier D. A Role for Apical Membrane Antigen 1 during Invasion of Hepatocytes by *Plasmodium falciparum* Sporozoites. *J. Biol. Chem.* 2004; 279: 9490-9496.

[31] Triglia T, Healer J, Caruana SR, Hodder AN, Anders RF, Crabb BS, Cowman AF. Apical membrane antigen 1 plays a central role in erythrocyte invasion by Plasmodium species. *Molecular Microbiology* 2000; 38: 706-718.

[32] Healer J, Crawford S, Ralph S, McFadden G, Cowman AF. Independent Translocation of Two Micronemal Proteins in Developing *Plasmodium falciparum* Merozoites. Infect. Immun. 2002; 70: 5751-5758.

[33] Howell SA, Withers-Martinez C, Kocken CH, Thomas AW, Blackman MJ. Proteolytic processing and primary structure of *Plasmodium falciparum* apical membrane antigen-1. *J. Biol. Chem.* 2001; 276: 31311-31320.

[34] Howell SA, Hackett F, Jongco AM, Withers-Martinez C, Kim K, Carruthers VB, Blackman MJ. Distinct mechanisms govern proteolytic shedding of a key invasion protein in apicomplexan pathogens. *Molecular Microbiology* 2005; 57: 1342-1356.

[35] Stowers AW, Kennedy MC, Keegan BP, Saul A, Long CA, Miller LH. Vaccination of Monkeys with Recombinant *Plasmodium falciparum* Apical Membrane Antigen 1 Confers Protection against Blood-Stage Malaria. Infect. Immun. 2002; 70: 6961-6967.

[36] Narum DL, Ogun SA, Thomas AW, Holder AA. Immunization with Parasite-Derived Apical Membrane Antigen 1 or Passive Immunization with a Specific Monoclonal Antibody Protects BALB/c Mice against Lethal *Plasmodium yoelii yoelii* YM Blood-Stage Infection. *Infect. Immun.* 2000; 68: 2899-2906.

[37] Coley AM, Gupta A, Murphy VJ, Bai T, Kim H, Anders RF, Foley M, Batchelor AH. Structure of the Malaria Antigen AMA1 in Complex with a Growth-Inhibitory Antibody. *PLoS Pathogens* 2007; 3: e138.

[38] Mueller MS, Renard A, Boato F, Vogel D, Naegeli M, Zurbriggen R, Robinson JA, Pluschke G. Induction of parasite growth-inhibitory antibodies by a virosomal formulation of a peptidomimetic of loop I from domain III of *Plasmodium falciparum* apical membrane antigen 1. *Infect. Immun.* 2003; 71: 4749-4758.

[39] Genton B, Pluschke G. A Randomized Placebo-Controlled Phase Ia Malaria Vaccine Trial of Two Virosome-Formulated Synthetic Peptides in Healthy Adult Volunteers. PLoS ONE 2007; 2: e1018.

[40] Okitsu SL, Silvie O, Westerfeld N, Curcic M, Kammer AR, Mueller MS, Sauerwein RW, Robinson JA, Genton B, Mazier D, Zurbriggen R, Pluschke G. A virosomal malaria Peptide vaccine elicits a long-lasting sporozoite-inhibitory antibody response in a phase 1a clinical trial. PLoS ONE 2007; 2: e1278.

[41] Kappe SHI, Buscaglia CA, Bergman LW, Coppens I, Nussenzweig V. Apicomplexan gliding motility and host cell invasion: overhauling the motor model. *Trends in Parasitology* 2004; 20: 13-16.

[42] Thompson FM, Porter DW, Okitsu SL, Westerfeld N, Vogel D, Todryk S, Poulton I, Correa S, Hutchings C, Berthoud T, Dunachie S, Andrews L, Williams JL, Sinden R, Gilbert SC, Pluschke G, Zurbriggen R, Hill AV. Evidence of Blood Stage Efficacy with a Virosomal Malaria Vaccine in a Phase IIa Clinical Trial. PLoS ONE 2008; 3: e1493.

[43] Okitsu SL, Boato F, Mueller MS, Li DB, Vogel D, Westerfeld N, Zurbriggen R, Robinson JA, Pluschke G. Antibodies elicited by a virosomally formulated *Plasmodium falciparum* serine repeat antigen-5 derived peptide detect the processed 47 kDa fragment both in sporozoites and merozoites. *Peptides* 2007; 28: 2051-2060.

[44] James S, Moehle K, Renard A, Mueller MS, Vogel D, Zurbriggen R, Pluschke G, Robinson JA. Synthesis, solution structure and immune recognition of an epidermal growth factor-like domain from *Plasmodium falciparum* merozoite surface protein-1. Chembiochem. 2006; 7: 1943-1950.

In: Immunologic Adjuvant Research
Editor: Antonio H. Benvenuto

ISBN 978-1-60692-399-3
© 2009 Nova Science Publishers, Inc.

Expert Commentary

Vaccine Adjuvants: Priorities and Challenges

Ali M. Harandi[4] *and Ole F. Olesen*[52]

1. Department of Microbiology and Immunology, Institute of Biomedicine, The Sahlgrenska Academy, University of Gothenburg, Sweden
2. Infectious Diseases Unit, DG Research, European Commission

"The views expressed are purely those of the writers and may not in any circumstances be regarded as stating an official position of the European Commission."

Abstract

The majority of vaccines presently under investigation represents highly pure recombinant proteins or subunits of pathogens and hence lacks most of the features of the original pathogens such as the inherent immunostimulatory property. Thus, the development of safe and potent immunologic adjuvants that can enhance and direct vaccine-specific immunity is urgently needed.

With few exceptions, aluminum hydroxide (alum) is currently the only vaccine adjuvant approved for human use worldwide. Although alum is effective at generating strong antibody response following repeated administration, it fails to elicit T cell immunity, which is essential to combat several life-threatening infections and cancers. This calls for rational design of prospective vaccine adjuvants that can establish protective immunity with fewer vaccinations with less injected material, through long-lasting antibody and cell-mediate immune responses. Recent developments in immunology, including the discovery of Toll-like receptors and other innate immune receptors with the capacity of bridging innate and adaptive immunity as well as novel delivery systems have offered new opportunities to delve into this avenue.

Despite the fact that the efficacy of new or improved vaccines depends critically on the accompanying adjuvants, research on vaccine adjuvants has so far received little

---

4 ali.harandi@microbio.gu.se
5 Ole.OLESEN@ec.europa.eu

attention as an independent scientific priority from most of the major research funding agencies and policy makers. At the same time, adjuvant research and development is currently spread over a wide number of highly diverse organizations, including large commercial companies, small biotech enterprises as well as publicly-funded research organizations and academia.

More efforts are therefore needed to highlight the importance of adjuvants on the global research agenda, but also to encourage collaboration and flow of information between different stakeholders. The European Commission has recognized the necessity to foster collaborative research, and has supported the development of novel or improved vaccines through successive Framework Programmes. Concurrent development and testing of new adjuvants has been an integrated part of these activities, and this has created a significant momentum in adjuvant research and development. Future challenges will be to keep up the momentum, to share available knowledge about adjuvants across sectors, and to facilitate access to the most promising adjuvants.

Introduction

Development and wide spread use of vaccines stand out as one of the public health interventions with the greatest impact on global health. Starting with the discovery of smallpox vaccine by Edward Jenner in the late 1700s, empirical approaches have been employed to develop vaccines against a variety of life-threatening infections in humans. Despite significant progress in this enterprise, vaccines to counter several life-threatening diseases especially those affecting the poor, including HIV/AIDS, malaria and tuberculosis as well as neglected infectious diseases are not available.

As a result of the significant reactogenicity problems associated with some traditional vaccines, the majority of vaccines presently under investigation represents highly pure recombinant or subunit of pathogens and hence lacks most of the features of the original pathogens such as the inherent immunostimulatory property. The shift away from traditional vaccines towards subunit vaccines demands the development of safe, potent immunologic adjuvants and delivery systems that can enhance and direct vaccine-specific immunity.

With few exceptions, aluminum hydroxide (alum) is currently the only vaccine adjuvant approved for human use worldwide. Although alum is effective at generating strong antibody response following repeated administration, some limitations of alum has become evident with continued human use. This includes the failure of alum in boosting immunizations with tetanus and diphtheria toxoids as well as influenza hemagglutinin antigen, lack of biodegradability combined with formation of granuloma at the injection site, as well as increases in immunoglobulin E response (Ott G and Van Nest G, 2007). Importantly, alum adjuvants are incapable of mounting T cell immunity, the type of immunity needed to combat several life-threatening infections and cancers. This calls for rational design of novel vaccine adjuvants that can establish protective immunity against different diseases through long-lasting antibody and cell-mediate immune responses.

Recent Developments and Future Challenges

Long after the introduction of alum, two potent new adjuvants were licensed for human use and this has led to recognition of adjuvants other than alum: MF59 (developed by Novartis) used in the flu vaccine Fluad®, and immunopotentiating reconstituted influenza virosome used in the hepatitis A vaccine Epaxal® (Berna Biotech). While MF59 showed satisfactory adjuvant effect with Fluad® (O'Hagan, DT, 2007), it had a limited adjuvant effect when used in conjunction with recombinant herpes simplex virus type 2 protein in a human vaccine trial carried out by Novartis (Stanberry LR, 2004). Moreover, MF59 did not appear to elicit potent cell mediated immunity.

Recent developments in immunology, including the discovery of Toll-like receptors (TLRs) and other innate immune receptors with the capacity of bridging innate and adaptive immunity have offered new opportunities. Promising advances have recently been made in the design of efficient adjuvants based on use of TLR agonists, and some TLR agonists reached advanced human trials. However, use of immunostimulatory molecules as immunopotentiators/vaccine adjuvants raises safety concerns, due to the likelihood of inducing overproduction of inflammatory molecules that may lead to induction of autoimmunity. Recently, human trials with Heplisav® (developed by Dynavax), which combines hepatitis B antigen with CpG sequence (ISS 1018), a TLR9 agonist, were halted in response to a serious adverse effect report from a phase 3 trial. After receiving two doses of Heplisav®, one of the vaccinees was preliminarily diagnosed with Wegener's granulomatosis, an autoimmune disease characterized by inflammation of the vasculature (DeFrancesco L, 2008). Monophosphoryl lipid A (MPL), a TLR4 agonist, is the only TLR-based adjuvant approved for human use. MPL in alum (AS04) is now as part of the hepatitis B virus (HBV) vaccine Fendrix®, and the human papiloma vaccine Cervarix® developed by GSK (Garçon N, 2007). Mode of action studies showed that TLR4 signaling for MPL is much biased towards the adaptor molecule Toll/interleukin-1 receptor-domain-containing adaptor protein inducing interferon β (TRIF), which generates no overt inflammation/reactogenicity in the host. This feature is unique to MPL as the natural TLR4 ligand LPS signals through the inflammatory adaptor proteins myeloid differentiation factor 88 (MyD88) as well as TRIF. It is noteworthy that a recent experimental study demonstrated that TLR signaling is dispensable for induction of antibody response by several standard adjuvants (Mata-Haro V et al, 2007). Based on the rapid evolution of this field it is likely that new generation of immunomodulatory adjuvants devoid of reactogenicity will be forthcoming.

Development of vaccine adjuvants suitable for mucosal administration represents another important challenge for vaccinologists. Although the majority of pathogens invade the body through or establish infection in the mucosal tissues, most vaccines licensed for human use are given parenterally. Mucosal vaccination has recently attracted much interest as a way of inducing protective mucosal as well as systemic immunity. Mucosal immunization offers certain advantages over the parenteral vaccine delivery, including less risk of transmitting certain type of infectious agents e.g., HIV and HBV and enhanced patient compliance due to ease of administration. Nonetheless, it has often proven difficult in practice to mount potent mucosal immunity and protection by mucosal administration of soluble protein antigens. In fact, only very few mucosal vaccines are presently approved for human use, including oral polio vaccine, the oral live-attenuated typhoid vaccine, oral cholera vaccines, an oral adenovirus vaccine (limited to military personnel), and an oral BCG strain used in Brazil (Holmgren, J et al, 2003). Recently, a nasal live attenuated flu vaccine (FluMist, MedImmune Vaccines, Inc.) has been approved for human use. It is thus becoming increasingly clear that the development of a broader range of mucosal vaccines demands development of safe yet effective mucosal adjuvants. Bacterial toxins such as cholera toxin (CT) and the closely analogous heat-labile enterotoxin (LT) and their derivatives are commonly used as potent mucosal adjuvants in experimental models; however, their toxicity has precluded their use for human vaccination. To circumvent toxicity, new generations of LT and CT mutants with reduced toxicity, and significant adjuvanticity have been developed among which LTK63 developed by Novartis reached advanced human trials. However, intranasal administration of toxin-based adjuvants is tied to an elevated risk of reactogenicity such as Bell's palsy in humans. The non toxic B subunit of CT (CTB) appeared to be safe for oral human use, and is now part of the licensed oral cholera vaccine Dukoral®; although, its capacity as mucosal adjuvant has proved to be limited (Holmgren J et al, 2003). Therefore, development of safe and potent mucosal adjuvants for human use is needed.

Numerous Fragmented Efforts

As more and more vaccines under development originate from modern molecular biology, the demand for safe and efficacious vaccine adjuvants is expected to increase dramatically. The available data on adjuvant safety and efficacy have mostly been generated using a wide variety of protocols, model systems and individual approaches, which makes it difficult or impossible to compare the activity of different adjuvants. At the moment, no comprehensive overview and comparative studies of adjuvants is therefore available. Each vaccine development project may therefore have to perform their own comparison of a large number of adjuvants in order to select the most efficacious ones. Such an exercise is both time-consuming and costly. This may result in the selection of a suboptimal adjuvant, which prevents the antigen from exercising its full potential and may eventually result in discontinuation of the vaccine development due to poor performance. The European Medicines Agency (EMEA) has recently issued "Guideline on adjuvants in vaccines for human use", which includes detailed directions for the testing of safety and efficacy of adjuvants for human use (EMEA/CHMP/VEG/134716/2004 Guideline on adjuvants in vaccines for human use, www.emea.europa.eu). Nonetheless, the establishment of a generally agreed set of standard tests for comparing different vaccine adjuvants remains an unmet need.

While use of novel vaccine adjuvants is attracting new attention from vaccine researchers, it is paradoxically difficult to access some of the promising new adjuvants for new vaccines. This can be attributed to the fragmented nature of adjuvant research, and the fact that many adjuvants are developed within large commercial organizations. Numerous proprietary adjuvants have thus been developed by the private sector, but these are only limited accessible to the public sector. For the private enterprises in possession of new adjuvants, providing them to third parties is often considered a commercial risk that could result in loss of competitive advantage and to the risk of adverse events happening in trials where new adjuvants are not properly used. As a consequence, many scientific data about adjuvants are not freely available in the public domain.

Many research projects on new vaccines against life threatening diseases such as malaria, TB and HIV as well as neglected tropical diseases has therefore been conducted with non-optimized adjuvants. This is particularly true for research and development carried out within the public sector or by small biotech companies. These organizations may be tempted to simply use aluminum salts that induce only antibody, or squalene-based water-in-oil emulsions which have safety and manufacturing issues. Such overly pragmatic approaches may result in otherwise viable antigens being abandoned as candidates for new vaccines, and consequently result in significant waste of resources from public and private domains.

The challenge is therefore to establish a system, which provides open access to adjuvants and adjuvant information to non-profit initiatives without affecting the freedom-of-operation of the owner of the adjuvant.

European and International Initiatives

The contribution of adjuvant research to vaccine development is largely underestimated, although an increasing awareness of the need for new adjuvants has dawned. Many organizations, private as well as public, are now participating in the search for new adjuvants. In spite of this, the major funding agencies for research in Europe and elsewhere have been slow to recognize adjuvant research as an independent scientific discipline, but a number of recent initiatives are trying to change this.

The European Adjuvant Advisory Committee (EAAC) was formed in 2003 to represent a large number of stakeholders with interests in adjuvant research. The EAAC comprises mostly biotech companies, and large vaccine manufacturers, but also a few academic groups (www.eaac.com). The EAAC was created to act as voice of consensus for those working in adjuvant research in Europe. It has the ambition to support the formation of a European research environment for adjuvants.

The Bill and Melinda Gates Foundation has recently awarded a grant to a Seattle-based Infectious Disease Research Institute to undertake a five-year project to develop and test new adjuvants. The project is mainly focusing on adjuvants for malaria vaccine candidates, but the results are likely to facilitate the development of vaccines against other infectious diseases as well.

The Global Adjuvant Development Initiative (GADI) was created in response to the need for public sector vaccine developers to have access to appropriate safe and effective adjuvants. GADI aims to provide the public-sector vaccine developers with adjuvants, knowledge on how to formulate these adjuvants and training on the formulation of vaccines. The objectives of GADI are to undertake the evaluation, comparison and development of adjuvants, and make the adjuvants available to the public sector.

The adjuvants and the knowledge and training related to adjuvant use that is being generated through GADI are being made available to the public sector through a network of vaccine development institutes and laboratories. This network, called AdjuNet is expected to facilitate the access to appropriate, safe and effective adjuvants to vaccine developers within public institution (university, government entity), multi-government entity, not-for-profit entities, and Product Development Partnerships (PDPs) (www.adjunet.net). GADI and AdjuNet are coordinated by the World Health Organization.

Within the European Union, vaccine research has been supported through national funding from the individual member states, as well as in a joint effort through the successive framework programmes of the European Commission (EC). In the recent 6th Framework Programme (FP6) for Research, the EC has initiated more than 60 collaborative projects on human vaccine research. Taken together, these projects gather more than 500 research groups from all over Europe and beyond, and with a total EC contribution of over €200 Mill to address a large number of research issues in basic vaccinology, translational vaccine research and clinical implementation of vaccines. Many of these projects include specific adjuvant research activities with an aim to test and develop new or improved adjuvants.

Some of these projects are already delivering important results that will contribute significantly to the advancement of knowledge about adjuvant research. One of the largest vaccine projects to be initiated during FP6 is the integrated project for new vaccines against tuberculosis (TB-VAC, www.TB-vac.org). This project gathers research groups from Europe and Africa in a common effort to develop new vaccines against tuberculosis, including the development of new subunit vaccines to replace or complement the existing live attenuated BCG vaccine. An integrated and essential component of the TB-VAC project is therefore also to identify the best adjuvant to accompany the subunit antigens in the clinical vaccine formulations.

The European Malaria Vaccine Development Association (EMVDA) is another integrated project, which aims to develop a vaccine for malaria. This project is to move candidate malaria antigen vaccines through pre-clinical and early clinical testing. One of the six work packages of this project is dedicated to adjuvant research and identification of the best suited adjuvant for a malaria vaccine (www.emvda.org).

While TB-VAC and EMVDA are focusing on systemic immunization approaches, the Mucosal Vaccines for Poverty Related Diseases (Muvapred) project is focusing on improved ways to elicit an efficient mucosal immune response. The objective of Muvapred is to advance the knowledge of mucosal vaccinology, with emphasis on a better understanding of mucosal adjuvants. This project has so far completed two clinical phase I trials with vaccines delivered through the nasal route. With another two clinical trials in preparation, the Muvapred consortium is expected to deliver valuable information on mucosal adjuvants and their mechanism of action (www.mucosalimmunity.org/muvapred).

Many of the European collaborative projects are thus providing important contributions to the advancement of adjuvant research. However, it is also clear that the adjuvant research activities are fragmented across several projects. Valuable information may therefore be lost if no mechanism exist to collect, coordinate and combine growing body of information and knowledge that are generated within individual projects.

Recently, the EC has therefore provided support to a new initiative, which aims to coordinate some of the ongoing activities for adjuvant research, both within Europe and globally. This project will provide a platform that comprises GADI, the EAAC and representatives from some of the major FP6 Integrated Projects (IP) in a common initiative called Pharvat. The aim of the project is to develop a comprehensive overview of existing and new adjuvants, compile a database of available information about these, and suggest methods that could be used to make a comparative testing of the safety and efficacy of adjuvants.

Conclusion

It is becoming increasingly evident that the efficacy of new vaccines depends critically on the accompanying adjuvants. In spite of this, the search for innovative adjuvants has so far received little attention as an independent scientific priority from most of the major research funding agencies and policy makers. At the same time, adjuvant research and development is currently spread over a wide number of highly diverse organizations, including large commercial companies, small biotech enterprises as well as publicly-funded research organizations and academia.

More efforts are therefore needed to highlight the importance of adjuvants on the global research agenda, but also to encourage collaboration and flow of information between the different stakeholders. The European Commission has recognized the necessity to foster collaborative research, and has supported the development of novel or improved vaccines through successive Framework Programmes. Concurrent development and testing of new adjuvants has been an integrated part of these activities, and this has created a significant momentum in adjuvant RandD. Future challenges will be to keep up the momentum, to pool available knowledge about adjuvants across sectors, and coordinate interaction between the global stakeholders and initiatives for adjuvant research.

References

DeFrancesco L. Dynavax trial halted, *Nature Biotechnology*, 2008, 26, 484.

Garçon N, Chomez P, Van Mechelen M. GlaxoSmithKline Adjuvant Systems in vaccines: concepts, achievements and perspectives. *Expert Rev. Vaccines*. 2007, 6, 723-39.

Gavin AL, Hoebe K, Duong B, Ota T, Martin C, Beutler B, Nemazee D. Adjuvant-enhanced antibody responses in the absence of toll-like receptor signaling. *Science,* 2006, 314, 1936-1938.

Holmgren J, Harandi AM, Czerkinsky C. Mucosal adjuvants and anti-infection and anti-immunopathology vaccines based on cholera toxin, cholera toxin B subunit and CpG DNA. *Expert Rev. Vaccines*. 2003, 2, 205-217.

Mata-Haro V, Cekic C, Martin M, Chilton PM, Casella CR, Mitchell TC. The vaccine adjuvant monophosphoryl lipid A as a TRIF-biased agonist of TLR4. *Science*. 2007, 316, 1628-1632.

O'Hagan DT. MF59 is a safe and potent vaccine adjuvant that enhances protection against influenza virus infection. *Expert Rev. Vaccines*. 2007, 6, 699-710.

Ott G and Van Nest G. Development of vaccine adjuvants - a historical perspective. Vaccine Adjuvants and Delivery Systems. Editor: Manmohan Singh. 2007; 1-32.

Stanberry LR. Clinical trials of prophylactic and therapeutic herpes simplex virus vaccines. Herpes. 2004, Suppl 3:161A-169A.

In: Immunologic Adjuvant Research
Editor: Antonio H. Benvenuto

ISBN 978-1-60692-399-3
© 2009 Nova Science Publishers, Inc.

Short Communication

The Involvement of Interleukin-6 in the Augmentation of Immune Response by Immunologic Adjuvants

Masahiko Mihara[6] *and Hiroto Yoshida*
Product Research Department, Chugai Pharmaceutical Co. Ltd.Japan

Abstract

In this article, we summarized studies that shed light on the involvement of IL-6 in immune reactions augmented by immunologic adjuvants such as complete Freund's adjuvant (CFA) and aluminum hydroxide (alum). Firstly, we considered humoral antibody responses. In one study, immunization with DNP-KLH plus CFA induced high blood IL-6 levels and augmented anti-DNP antibody production compared with DNP-KLH alone. Blockade of IL-6 signaling by anti-IL-6 receptor (IL-6R) antibody dose-dependently suppressed the increase in CFA-augmented anti-DNP antibody production. In another study, immunization with OVA plus alum augmented anti-OVA IgE production, but IL-6 production was not detectable and anti-IL-6R antibody did not suppress IgE production. Secondly, we considered cellular immune responses. Delayed-type hypersensitivity (DTH), an antigen-specific, cell-mediated immune reaction, was elicited by CFA plus antigen. Spleen cells from immunized mice produced IL-2 and IFN-γ when stimulated by antigen (mycobacteria), suggesting that CFA induces Th1 differentiation. Anti-IL-6R antibody significantly suppressed the DTH reaction and the production of IL-2 and IFN-γ by spleen cells, suggesting that IL-6 is needed for the DTH reaction and for Th1 differentiation. Th17, a recently discovered helper T cell that produces IL-17, is attracting attention for its role in autoimmune disease models. To study this, collagen-induced arthritis (CIA) was induced by two immunizations with type II collagen plus CFA. Th1 cells and Th17 cells were induced in spleen in this model. When injected at the first immunization, anti-IL-6R antibody suppressed the onset of

---

[6] Address correspondence and reprint requests to Masahiko Mihara, Ph.D. Chugai Pharmaceutical Co. Ltd., 135, Komakado 1-chome, Gotemba-shi, Shizuoka, 412-8513, Japan, Phone: 81-550-87-6739, Fax: 81-550-87-6782, Email: miharamsh@chugai-pharm.co.jp.

arthritis and the induction of Th1 and Th17 cells. In conclusion, IL-6 plays a crucial role in CFA-augmented immune reactions, but not in alum-augmented ones. Since CFA and alum evoke different immune responses, and this should be taken into account when using them as adjuvants.

1. Introduction

An adjuvant is an agent that stimulates the immune system, increasing its response to antigens. Freund's adjuvant and aluminum hydroxide (alum) are widely used as adjuvants in animal studies. Complete Freund's adjuvant (CFA) is an water-in-oil emulsion containing inactivated and dried mycobacteria, usually *Mycobacterium tuberculosis*. CFA is effective in stimulating humoral antibody response and cellular immune response. Alum also stimulates strong humoral antibody response, for which reason it is included as an adjuvant in some vaccines.

Animal models established by immunization with antigen plus adjuvant are important for the study of disease processes in, and potential therapies for, autoimmune diseases. To understand these models fully, the involvement of cytokines in the activation of humoral and cellular immune responses by adjuvants needs to be better understood.

It is particularly important to understand the involvement of interleukin-6 (IL-6) in the activation of this response because it is a multifunctional cytokine that plays essential roles in host defense mechanisms through its involvement in the immune system and in hematopoiesis. IL-6 induces antibody production by differentiating activated B cells into antibody-producing cells, stimulates the proliferation of peripheral T cells and mature thymocytes, and induces differentiation of cytotoxic T cells [1].

In this article, therefore, we summarize the findings of studies that we have conducted that shed light on the involvement of IL-6 in immune responses augmented by the immunologic adjuvants, CFA and alum.

2. Humoral Antibody Responses

2.1. Humoral Response by CFA

CFA is widely used as an adjuvant when immunizing animals with antigens because it induces higher antibody titers. Its adjuvant activity results from its sustained release with the antigen from oily emulsion and its stimulation of local immune responses.

In an earlier article [2], we described the role of IL-6 in antibody production when an antigen was immunized in combination with CFA. In that study, C3H/HeJ mice were immunized intraperitoneally with dinitrophenol (DNP)-keyhole limpet hemocyanin (KLH) plus CFA or DNP-KLH plus saline on day 0. Rat anti-mouse IL-6R antibody (MR16-1) was injected intraperitoneally immediately after immunization (day 0) and again on days 2 and 5. Serum anti-DNP antibody levels were measured on days 7 and 14 using a DNP-BSA-coated ELISA plate.

Administration of DNP-KLH with CFA caused significantly higher anti-DNP antibody production than administration of DNP-KLH with saline, so CFA was an effective adjuvant in this model. Serum IL-6 was detectable in the antigen/CFA group (25.3 pg/mL on day 7; 3.2 pg/mL on day 14), but not in the antigen/saline group, suggesting that CFA induced IL-6 production. Administration of MR16-1 significantly suppressed the augmentation of anti-DNP antibody production by CFA (Figure 1), which clearly shows that CFA-induced IL-6 plays an important role in the augmentation of antibody production by CFA. This hypothesis is also supported by the fact that exogenous IL-6 injection augmented antibody production in mice immunized with DNP-KLH in saline [3].

Since IL-6 was originally discovered as a factor that differentiates activated B cells into antibody-producing cells [4] and CFA is a potent inducer of IL-6 production, it is not surprising that the augmentation of antibody production by CFA is mediated by CFA-induced IL-6.

2.2. Humoral Response by Alum

Alum stimulates good antibody response. It is particularly effective as an adjuvant to augment IgE production [5]. We therefore conducted a study to examine the effect of IL-6 blockade on antigen-IgE production induced by antigen plus alum.

C3H/HeJ mice were immunized intraperitoneally with ovalbumin (OVA) plus alum on day 0 and then boosted on day 21. Serum was collected on day 35 and total IgE, anti-OVA IgE and anti-OVA IgG were measured by ELISA. MR16-1 was injected on day 0 (immediately after immunization) and on days 2 and 5. Total IgE, anti-OVA IgE and anti-OVA IgG production were clearly augmented by OVA plus alum, but not alum alone. The administration of MR16-1 did not affect the production of these antibodies (Figure 2).

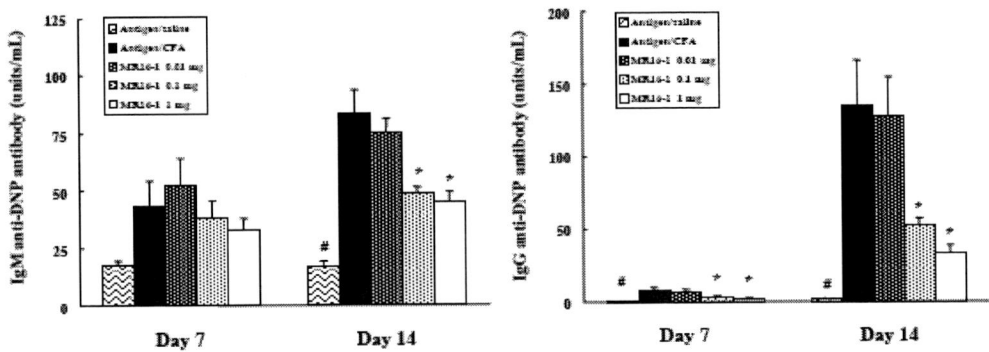

Female C3H/HeJ mice were immunized i.p. with DNP-KLH in CFA on day 0. MR16-1 was injected i.p. on days 0, 2, and 5. Blood was collected on days 7 and 14. Serum anti-DNP antibody levels were measured by ELISA. Columns and error bars show the mean and S.E. of 5 mice. Statistical significances between the antigen/saline and antigen/CFA groups, and between the antigen/CFA and MR16-1 groups were analyzed by the unpaired t test ($^{\#}P<0.05$) and the Dunnett's multiple comparison test (*$P<0.05$), respectively.

Figure 1. CFA-augmented antibody production was inhibited by anti-IL-6R antibody.

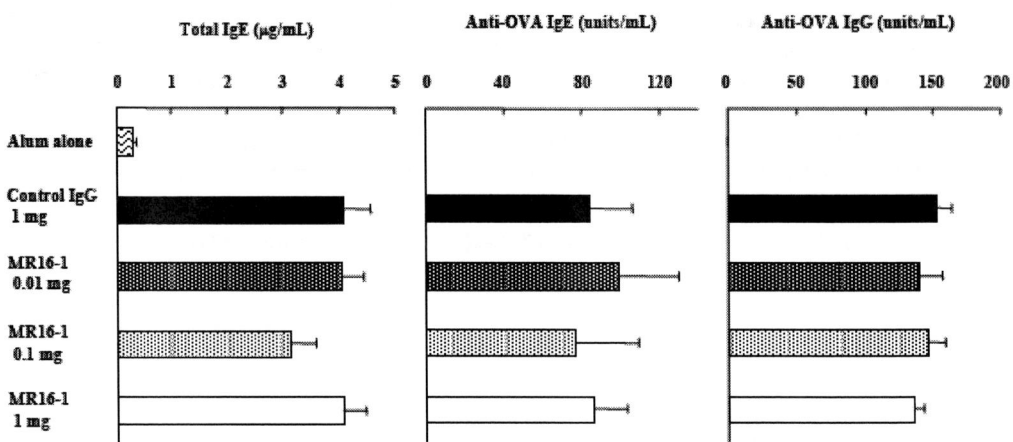

Female C3H/HeJ mice were immunized i.p. with OVA plus alum on day 0, and boosted on day 21. MR16-1 was injected i.p. on days 0, 2, and 5. The mice were bled on day 35, and serum total IgE, anti-OVA IgE and anti-OVA IgG levels were measured by ELISA. Columns and error bars show the mean and S.E. of 5 mice.

Figure 2. Alum-augmented IgE production was not inhibited by anti-IL-6R antibody.

Moreover, treatment with MR16-1 after the booster on day 21 did not suppress antibody production. IL-6 was not detected in serum from any of the groups.

Taken together, the results of this study demonstrate that IL-6 is not involved in IgE production induced by immunization with antigen plus alum. On the other hand, it has been reported that alum-augmented IgE production is inhibited by anti-IL-4 antibody, indicating that IL-4 is an essential cytokine for alum-augmented IgE production [6,7].

3. Cellular Responses

3.1. DTH Response

CFA also stimulates cellular immune response, including Delayed-type hypersensitivity (DTH) reactions. DTH reactions are antigen-specific, cell-mediated, immune responses. Cutaneous DTH reactions are initiated when $CD4^+$ memory T cells are activated by Langerhans cells and other antigen-presenting cells in the skin. Upon activation, these $CD4^+$ T cells release inflammatory mediators that recruit effector cells to the site of the antigen challenge. Monocytes/macrophages are thought to be the main effector cells, but $CD8^+$ T cells and natural-killer (NK) cells are also thought to participate in DTH reactions. The tuberculin skin reaction is a classic DTH reaction.

The role of IL-6 in DTH reactions was investigated in another part of the study mentioned above [2]. Mice were immunized with CFA containing heat-killed mycobacteria (*Mycobacterium butyricum*). Fourteen days later, antigen was injected into the footpads of the mice. Footpad swelling was measured 24 hours after this antigen challenge.

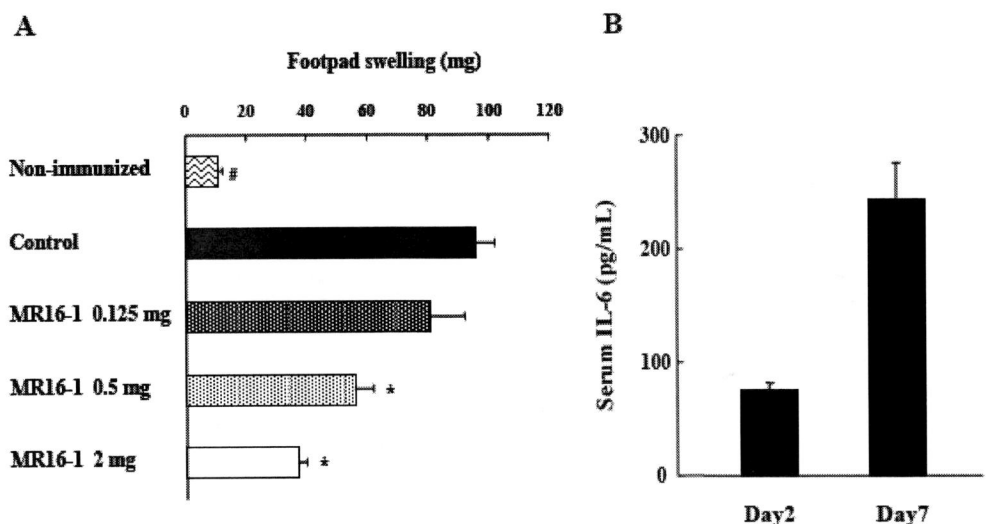

MR16-1 was administered i.p. on the day of immunization (Day 0). Antigen was injected on day 14. (A) Footpad swelling 24 hours after antigen challenge. (B) Serum IL-6 in control immunized mice on days 2 and 7. Each column and error bar indicates the mean ± S.E. of 5 mice. For (A), statistical significances between the non-immunized group and the control group, and between the control group and the MR16-1 groups, were analyzed by the unpaired t test ($^{\#}$ P<0.05) and the Dunnett's multiple comparison test (*P<0.05), respectively.

Figure 3. Mycobacteria-induced DTH reaction was suppressed by MR16-1.

A single injection of MR16-1 immediately after immunization significantly suppressed footpad swelling (Figure 3A), and elevation of serum IL-6 levels were observed in control immunized mice (Fig 3B). These findings suggest that IL-6 plays an important role in the DTH response.

Since it is known that the DTH response is mediated by Th1 cells [8], we conducted an *in vitro* examination of the antigen-specific production of Th1-type cytokines (IL-2 and IFN-γ) from spleen cells obtained from the above mice. Production of IL-2 and IFN-γ was undetectable for normal mice, considerable for control immunized mice and marginal for MR16-1-treated immunized mice [2]. These findings suggest that IL-6 is important for the production of the Th1-type cytokines that mediate the DTH response.

3.2. CIA

Collagen-induced arthritis (CIA) is an experimental autoimmune arthritis model that is widely used for studying disease processes in, and potential therapies for, rheumatoid arthritis [9].

In a study conducted to investigate the role of IL-6 in CIA [10], DBA/1J mice were immunized with bovine type II collagen (CII) emulsified with CFA and then boosted 3 weeks later.

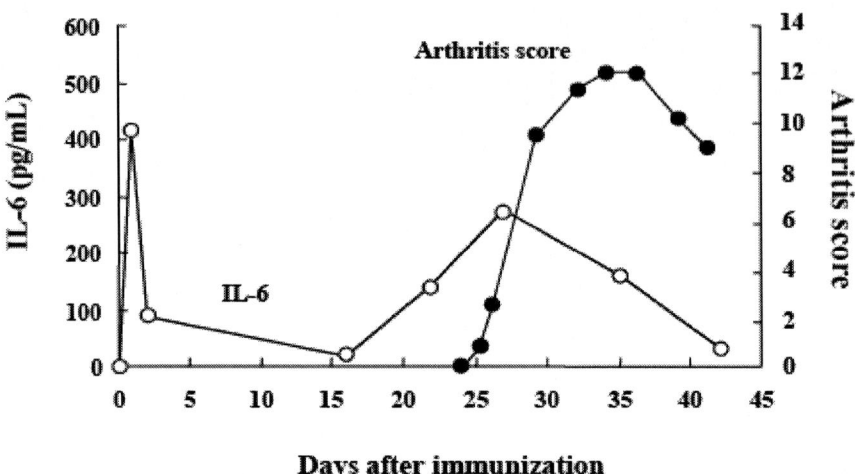

Bovine CII emulsified with CFA was injected on days 0 and 21. Serum IL-6 was measured by ELISA. The arthritis score was determined by evaluating arthritis symptoms in all 4 limbs using a visual scoring system.

Figure 4. Serum IL-6 levels in a mouse CIA model.

IL-6 production was induced within 24 hours after the first CII immunization and then decreased rapidly. After the booster injection on day 21, serum IL-6 levels increased again and decreased slowly (Figure 4). The slower decrease may be due to the onset of arthritis.

MR16-1 inhibited the onset of arthritis when it was injected immediately after the first CII immunization, but not when it was injected immediately after the second CII immunization. These results suggest that, in this CIA model, the increase in IL-6 after the first immunization is very important for the onset of arthritis, whereas the increase in IL-6 after the second immunization is not.

CFA has been widely used in the induction of several animal models of autoimmune diseases. It is known that $CD4^+$ helper T cells consist of two subsets, Th1 cells and Th2 cells, largely on the basis of the cytokines they produce [11]. Recently, another population of $CD4^+$ T cells has been described, namely Th17 cells, which are characterized by the production of IL-17 [12]. The role of Th17 cells in autoimmune pathology is now becoming recognized, interestingly in events that were previously thought to be Th1-mediated.

In another study, we examined the induction of Th1 and Th17 cells in CIA models by the production of IFN-γ and IL-17, respectively, by splenic $CD4^+$ T cells. Mice were immunized with CII emulsified in CFA and injected with MR16-1. Three weeks later, $CD4^+$ T cells purified from spleen cells from those mice were re-stimulated *in vitro* with CII for 48 hours in the presence of anti-CD28 antibody. After culture, IFN-γ and IL-17 concentrations in the supernatant were measured. Production of IFN-γ and IL-17 was negligible for non-immunized mice, abundant for control immunized mice, and significantly less for MR16-1-treated immunized mice (Figure 5). The production of IFN-γ and IL-17 in cells from CIA mice suggests that Th1 cells and Th17 cells were both induced by immunization with CII plus CFA.

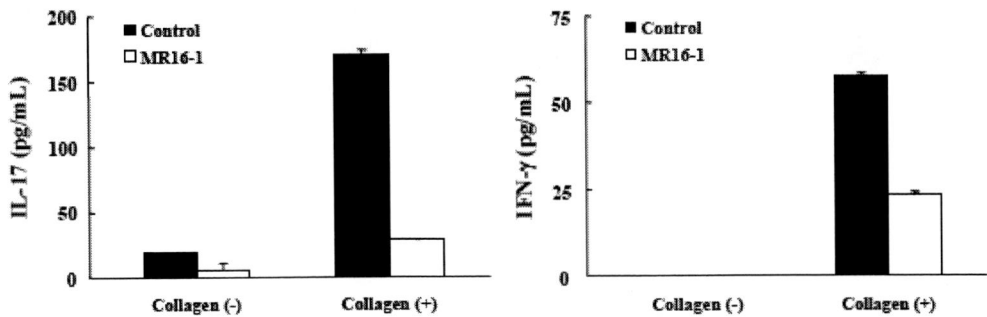

CD4 T cells purified from the spleen of CIA mice were cultured with Bovine CII and anti-CD28 antibody for 48 hours. After culture, IL-17 and IFN-g production were measured.

Figure 5. Production of IL-17 and IFN-γ by splenic CD4 T cells from CIA mice.

The decreased production of these cytokines in cells from MR16-1-treated mice shows that IL-6 made a major contribution to the production of IFN-γ and IL-17, suggesting that IL-6 may contribute to the differentiation of Th1 and Th17 cells in vivo.

Naïve T cells differentiate into Th17 cells when stimulated with antigen in the presence of both IL-6 and TGF-β in an *in vitro* study using mouse cells [13,14], so it is likely that Th17 cell differentiation was inhibited by IL-6 blockade at the time of immunization.

By contrast, the involvement of IL-6 in Th1 cell differentiation is controversial. It has been reported that IL-6 inhibits Th1 cell differentiation [15]. Conversely, it has been reported that Th1 response can be suppressed by IL-6 blockade [16,17], as we found in our study, implying that IL-6 may be necessary for Th1 cell differentiation. Further studies seem to be needed to clarify this issue.

8. Conclusions

In relation to humoral antibody responses, IL-6 plays a central role in CFA-augmented antibody production, but not in alum-augmented antibody production.

In relation to cellular immune responses, IL-6 is strongly involved in CFA-augmented responses such as the DTH response and CIA by differentiating naïve CD4$^+$ cells into Th17 and Th1 cells.

Since CFA and alum evoke different immune responses, this should be taken into account when using them as adjuvants.

9. References

[1] Akira, S; Taga, T; Kishimoto T. Interleukin-6 in biology and medicine. *Adv. Immunol.* 1993;54:2-78.

[2] Mihara, M; Nishimoto, N; Yoshizaki, K; Suzuki, T. Influences of anti-mouse interleukin-6 receptor antibody on immune responses in mice. *Immunol. Lett.* 2002;84:223-229.

[3] Okazaki, M; Yamada, Y; Nishimoto, N; Yoshizaki, K; Mihara, M. Characterization of anti-mouse interleukin-6 receptor antibody. *Immunol. Lett* 2002;84:231-240.

[4] Muraguchi, A; Hirano, T; Tang, B; Matsuda, T; Horii, Y; Nakajima, K; Kishimoto, T. The essential role of B cell stimulatory factor 2 (BSF-2/IL-6) for the terminal differentiation of B cells. *J. Exp. Med* 1988;167:332-344.

[5] Kudo, K; Okudaira, H; Miyamoto, T; Nakagawa, T; Horiuchi, Y. IgE antibody response to mite antigen in the mouse. Suppression of an established IgE antibody response by chemically modified antigen. *J. Allergy Clin. Immunol.* 1978;61:1-9.

[6] Finkelman, FD; Katona, IM; Urban, JF Jr; Paul, WE. Control of in vivo IgE production in the mouse by interleukin 4. *Ciba Found Symp.* 1989;147:3-17.

[7] Takenaka, T; Kuribayashi, K; Nakamine, H; Tsujimoto, M; Fukuhara, Y; Maeda, J; Mihara, M; Uchiyama, Y; Ohsugi, Y. Regulation by cytokines of eosinophilopoiesis and immunoglobulin E production in mice. *Immunology* 1993;78:541-546.

[8] Cher, DJ; Mosmann, TR. Two types of murine helper T cell clone. II. Delayed-type hypersensitivity is mediated by TH1 clones. *J. Immunol.* 1987;138:3688-3694.

[9] Trentham, DE; Townes, AS; Kang, AH. Autoimmunity to type II collagen: an experimental model of arthritis. *J. Exp. Med.* 1977;146:857-868.

[10] Takagi, N; Mihara, M; Moriya, Y; Nishimoto, N; Yoshizaki, K; Kishimoto, T; Takeda, Y; Ohsugi, Y. Blockage of interleukin-6 receptor ameliorates joint disease in murine collagen-induced arthritis. *Arthritis Rheum.* 1998;41:2117-2121.

[11] Mosmann, TR; Coffman, RL. TH1 and TH2 cells: different patterns of lymphokine secretion lead to different functional properties. *Annu. Rev. Immunol.* 1989;7:145-173

[12] Harrington, LE; Hatton, RD; Mangan, PR; Turner, H; Murphy, TL; Murphy, KM; Weaver, CT. Interleukin 17-producing CD4+ effector T cells develop via a lineage distinct from the T helper type 1 and 2 lineages. *Nat. Immunol.* 2005;6:1123-1132.

[13] Bettelli, E; Carrier, Y; Gao, W; Korn, T; Strom, TB; Oukka, M; Weiner, HL; Kuchroo, VK. Reciprocal developmental pathways for the generation of pathogenic effector TH17 and regulatory T cells. *Nature* 2006;441:235-238.

[14] Veldhoen, M; Hocking, RJ; Atkins, CJ; Locksley, RM; Stockinger, B. TGFbeta in the context of an inflammatory cytokine milieu supports de novo differentiation of IL-17-producing T cells. *Immunity* 2006;24:179-189.

[15] Diehl, S; Anguita, J; Hoffmeyer, A; Zapton, T; Ihle, JN; Fikrig, E; Rincón, M. Inhibition of Th1 differentiation by IL-6 is mediated by SOCS1. *Immunity* 2000;13:805-815.

[16] Yamamoto, M; Yoshizaki, K; Kishimoto, T; Ito, H. IL-6 is required for the development of Th1 cell-mediated murine colitis. *J. Immunol.* 2000;164:4878-4882.

[17] Okuda, Y; Sakoda, S; Bernard, CC; Fujimura, H; Saeki, Y; Kishimoto, T; Yanagihara, T. IL-6-deficient mice are resistant to the induction of experimental autoimmune encephalomyelitis provoked by myelin oligodendrocyte glycoprotein. *Int. Immunol.* 1998;10:703-708.

Index

A

abdominal, 76
aberrant, 4, 31
abnormalities, 34
absorption, 77, 96
academic, 103
access, 100, 102, 103
accounting, 75
acid, 8, 15, 19, 50, 57, 58, 67, 71, 91, 92
acquired immunity, 71
acquired immunodeficiency syndrome, 20
actin, 22
activation, 1, 6, 7, 11, 12, 16, 18, 21, 22, 26, 28, 49, 51, 52, 53, 54, 55, 56, 57, 59, 60, 61, 62, 63, 64, 65, 66, 67, 69, 71, 90, 91, 96, 108, 110
acute, 22, 59, 65
acute leukemia, 22
adaptive immune system, 5, 7, 20, 49, 51, 54, 90, 91
adenocarcinoma, 37, 38, 41
adenocarcinomas, 32
adenovirus, 102
adhesion, 4, 35, 55
administration, 12, 16, 21, 22, 23, 39, 41, 42, 43, 70, 73, 75, 77, 83, 99, 100, 101, 109
adsorption, 40
adults, 39, 72
adverse event, 15, 16, 17, 93, 102
aerosol, 17
Africa, 92, 104
Ag, 2, 13
agent, 1, 3, 22, 108
agents, 3, 8, 49, 56, 58, 62, 101
aging, 13

agonist, 57, 59, 60, 69, 70, 71, 72, 101, 105
airway hyperresponsiveness, 70
Alberta, 31
allergens, 75, 81
allergic, 59, 60, 70, 71, 72, 74, 85
allergic asthma, 59, 70
allergic inflammation, 74
allergic reaction, 60
allergic rhinitis, 72
allergy, 18, 60
allogeneic, 22, 23, 27, 28, 29, 36, 39, 40, 42, 45
alpha, 41, 69, 71
alternative, 13, 23, 24, 28, 40, 54
aluminium, 8, 11, 12, 36, 44, 45
aluminum, 2, 8, 9, 11, 12, 13, 35, 38, 44, 49, 99, 100, 103, 107, 108
amelioration, 70
amino, 51, 58, 69, 90, 92, 93
amino acid, 51, 90, 92, 93
analog, 68, 69
angiogenesis, 69, 86
animal models, 4, 14, 18, 22, 26, 31, 58, 112
animal studies, 58, 108
animals, 25, 26, 29, 33, 108
anorexia, 21
anti-apoptotic, 54
anti-bacterial, 50
antibiotic, 62
antibodies, 41, 47, 92, 94, 95, 98
antibody, 2, 5, 6, 11, 12, 14, 17, 19, 31, 32, 33, 35, 37, 43, 44, 59, 60, 77, 78, 81, 82, 89, 90, 92, 93, 98, 99, 100, 101, 103, 105, 107, 108, 109, 110, 112, 113, 114

anti-cancer, 1, 17, 40, 43, 58
anti-gas, 19
antigen, 1, 2, 3, 4, 5, 6, 7, 8, 9, 10, 11, 12, 13, 15, 17, 21, 22, 23, 26, 27, 30, 31, 32, 33, 35, 36, 38, 39, 41, 42, 43, 44, 45, 46, 47, 49, 50, 57, 60, 72, 73, 74, 77, 78, 79, 83, 84, 85, 89, 90, 91, 93, 95, 96, 97, 98, 100, 101, 102, 104, 107, 108, 109, 110, 111, 113, 114
antigen presenting cells (APCs), 1, 4, 5, 7, 21, 46, 49, 50, 57, 74, 77, 91, 92, 110
anti-idiotypic, 11, 35, 37
anti-inflammatory, 46
antimicrobial, 50, 54
antimicrobial protein, 50
antitumor, 22, 26, 36, 38, 42, 44, 45, 59, 66, 68, 85
anti-tumor, 1, 3, 5, 6, 7, 16, 19, 20, 22, 26, 27, 28, 35, 37, 66, 73, 74, 79, 83
apoptosis, 5, 6, 7, 55, 64, 67
apoptotic, 5, 6, 54, 67
apoptotic effect, 5, 6
application, 13, 15, 27, 73, 77, 78, 79, 81, 82, 84, 87
arginine, 8
arthritis, 55, 107, 111, 112, 114
asexual, 93, 94
asthma, 18, 59, 60, 70, 71, 74, 87
atopic dermatitis, 74, 85, 86, 87
atopic eczema, 87
attachment, 16, 90
attention, 15, 100, 102, 105, 107
Austria, 1
autoantibody, 70
autocrine, 66
autoimmune, 2, 101, 107, 108, 111, 112, 114
autoimmune disease, 101, 107, 108, 112
autoimmunity, 9, 29, 34, 59, 70, 101
availability, 28, 90
awareness, 103

B

B cell, 4, 5, 6, 15, 20, 21, 51, 60, 66, 71, 90, 91, 92, 94, 108, 109, 114
B cells, 5, 6, 21, 51, 60, 71, 91, 92, 108, 109, 114
bacillus, 8, 16, 17, 23, 46
bacteria, 16, 18, 19, 21, 57, 58
bacterial, 3, 6, 8, 9, 10, 15, 18, 19, 31, 42, 49, 50, 51, 57, 58, 59, 60, 61, 67, 69, 71, 73, 74, 84
bacterial infection, 6, 42, 61

barrier, 75, 76, 77, 81, 83, 85
basal cell carcinoma, 59
B-cell, 54, 73, 74, 95
BCG vaccine, 46, 104
bell, 27
bell-shaped, 27
beneficial effect, 26
benefits, 12, 30, 46
beta, 63, 65
bias, 18
binding, 8, 11, 16, 20, 34, 35, 52, 54, 58, 91, 92, 94, 95
biochemical, 80
biochemistry, 68
biodegradability, 100
biodegradable, 8, 24, 26, 38
biologic, 11
biological, 14, 20, 22, 36, 63, 65, 66, 67, 68, 69, 71, 90, 96
biological activity, 36
biologically, 56
biology, 20, 61, 62, 63, 70, 102, 113
biomarkers, 61
biomimetic, 43
biopharmaceuticals, 1, 13
biophysical, 96
bladder, 16, 37, 46
bladder cancer, 16, 46
blocks, 95
blood, 7, 11, 13, 30, 55, 61, 64, 91, 93, 94, 95, 107
blood monocytes, 11
blot, 94
B-lymphocytes, 21
bolus, 21, 39, 43
bonding, 93
bonds, 60
bone, 30, 39, 59, 65, 70
bone marrow, 39, 59, 65, 70
Boston, 49
bovine, 111
Brazil, 102
breast, 4, 14, 31, 32, 38, 39, 41, 42, 43
breast cancer, 14, 32, 38, 41, 42, 43
building blocks, 95
bystander cells, 28

C

calcium, 9, 12, 36, 38, 40

Canada, 10, 17, 31
cancer, 1, 2, 3, 4, 7, 9, 10, 11, 13, 14, 15, 16, 17, 18, 19, 20, 21, 22, 23, 24, 28, 29, 30, 31, 32, 33, 35, 36, 37, 38, 39, 40, 41, 42, 43, 44, 45, 46, 47, 51, 54, 56, 59, 60, 61, 62, 63, 68, 69, 70, 71, 86
cancer cells, 4, 31, 33, 40
cancer progression, 54
cancer treatment, 31
cancers, ix, 4, 19, 31, 44, 99, 100
candidates, 35, 43, 49, 51, 89, 93, 103
capacity, 2, 20, 83, 93, 99, 101, 102
carbohydrate, 2, 4, 7, 8, 12, 17, 31, 32, 35, 40
carboxyl, 69
carcinoembryonic antigen, 4
carcinogenicity, 59
carcinoma, 16, 20, 21, 23, 26, 29, 37, 40, 42, 43, 44, 46, 59, 68
carcinomas, 35, 43, 44
cardiovascular, 21, 69
carrier, 12, 19, 33, 35, 90, 91, 96
caspase, 55, 64
catalytic, 54, 84
CD14, 13, 55, 58, 64, 65, 68
CD19, 87
CD1d, 27
CD28, 112, 113
CD34, 70
CD34+, 70
CD4, 3, 5, 6, 7, 19, 21, 26, 27, 28, 36, 66, 74, 82, 84, 86, 87, 91, 95, 96, 110, 112, 113, 114
CD40, 6, 21, 54, 57, 66
CD8+, 5, 6, 7, 26, 27, 28, 42, 44, 45, 110
CDC, 5, 6
CDK4, 4
cell, 1, 3, 4, 5, 6, 7, 8, 10, 11, 13, 14, 15, 17, 18, 20, 21, 22, 23, 24, 26, 27, 28, 29, 30, 34, 35, 36, 37, 38, 39, 40, 41, 42, 43, 44, 45, 46, 50, 51, 54, 55, 57, 59, 60, 61, 62, 63, 64, 66, 67, 70, 71, 74, 78, 79, 80, 82, 84, 85, 86, 87, 90, 91, 92, 94, 95, 96, 98, 99, 100, 101, 107, 110, 113, 114
cell adhesion, 4, 35
cell cycle, 4
cell differentiation, 60, 78, 113
cell growth, 21, 55
cell invasion, 92, 94, 98
cell line, 23, 28, 29, 30, 43, 45, 55, 94
cell surface, 4, 57, 64, 91
cell transplantation, 36

cellular immunity, 8, 74, 94
central nervous system, 21
cervical, 4, 37
cervical cancer, 4
cervical carcinoma, 37
CFA, 107, 108, 109, 110, 111, 112, 113
Chávez, 85
chemical, 8, 14, 43, 90, 91
chemistry, 63, 65, 67, 68, 69, 71
chemoattractants, 44
chemokine, 55, 56, 61, 64
chemokine receptor, 55, 64
chemokines, 13, 54, 56, 57, 80, 81, 85
chemotaxis, 55
chemotherapy, 19, 32, 39, 61, 69
children, 11
cholera, 8, 19, 38, 45, 102, 105
cholesterol, 15
choriocarcinoma, 45
chorionic gonadotropin, 4
chromatography, 68
chronic, 3, 21, 59, 70, 80
chronic lymphocytic leukemia, 59
chronic myelogenous, 21
classes, 18, 60
classical, 16
classified, 80
clinical, 2, 3, 9, 11, 12, 14, 15, 16, 17, 19, 20, 21, 22, 23, 26, 27, 28, 29, 30, 33, 34, 36, 37, 40, 41, 42, 44, 45, 49, 60, 61, 62, 71, 72, 79, 93, 94, 95, 98, 104
clinical trial, 9, 11, 12, 15, 16, 17, 19, 23, 26, 27, 30, 37, 49, 93, 94, 95, 98, 104
clone, 114
clones, 84, 114
Co, 58, 62, 77, 107
codes, 38
coding, 39
colitis, 114
collaboration, 100, 105
collagen, 107, 111, 114
colloidal particles, 15
colon, 16, 32, 38, 39, 46
colon cancer, 16, 32, 38, 39, 46
colony-stimulating factor, 8, 22, 26, 36, 37, 41, 44, 45
colorectal, 4, 16, 19, 20, 23, 31, 35, 39, 41, 42, 43, 44, 46
colorectal cancer, 19, 20, 35, 39, 41, 42, 44
combat, 99, 100

commercial, 12, 40, 100, 102, 105
competitive advantage, 102
complement, 5, 6, 31, 35, 104
complexity, 96
compliance, 101
complications, 16
components, 3, 11, 49, 51, 53, 54, 57, 67, 91, 94, 95
compounds, 12, 38, 63, 75, 77
concentration, 70
conditioning, 91
conformational, 52, 90
conformational states, 90
conjugation, 90
consensus, 103
conservation, 51, 92
construction, 14
control, 3, 25, 29, 32, 36, 54, 56, 61, 65, 66, 74, 81, 82, 93, 94, 111, 112
control group, 25, 32, 93, 111
controlled, 16, 19, 26, 39, 41, 44, 83
correlation, 30
cost-effective, 74, 77, 83, 90
costimulatory molecules, 4, 5, 7, 11, 57
costimulatory signal, 6, 7
coupling, 35, 40, 63
covering, 92
COX-2, 73, 77, 78, 79, 80, 83
COX-2 inhibitors, 79
critical analysis, 42
cross-linking, 91
cryosurgery, 59, 70
crystal, 93
crystal structure, 93
crystals, 43
C-terminal, 51, 54
C-terminus, 91
culture, 13, 58, 112, 113
cutaneous T-cell lymphoma, 21
CXCL8, 13
cyclooxygenase, 86, 87
cyclooxygenase-2, 86, 87
cyclophosphamide, 32, 42
cytokine, 1, 2, 3, 5, 7, 10, 11, 12, 15, 16, 21, 23, 24, 26, 28, 33, 35, 37, 38, 39, 40, 42, 46, 53, 59, 60, 61, 69, 77, 78, 80, 82, 84, 108, 110, 114
cytokine response, 15, 69
cytokines, 2, 3, 5, 6, 7, 8, 14, 16, 20, 22, 23, 24, 26, 28, 35, 36, 37, 46, 49, 54, 56, 57, 60, 73, 74, 77, 80, 81, 82, 83, 85, 91, 108, 111, 112, 113, 114
cytoplasm, 54
cytoplasmic tail, 51
cytosine, 85
cytosol, 7, 20, 91
cytosolic, 38, 55
cytotoxic, 6, 7, 11, 13, 16, 19, 22, 42, 43, 61, 66, 74, 84, 92, 96, 108
cytotoxicity, 5, 6, 35, 40, 83

D

danger, 4, 7, 8, 18, 41
database, 105
de novo, 26, 114
death, 6, 53, 87
defense, 63, 108
defense mechanisms, 63, 108
deficiency, 81
definition, 2
degradation, 8, 53, 54, 69, 90
degree, 12
delays, 64
delivery, 8, 15, 23, 24, 26, 40, 74, 77, 78, 89, 91, 92, 93, 94, 95, 96, 97, 99, 100, 101
Delta, 59
demand, 3, 102
dendritic cell, 4, 7, 13, 19, 21, 22, 27, 30, 36, 38, 44, 49, 50, 51, 56, 57, 63, 66, 67, 70, 71, 73, 74, 84, 86, 87
density, 40
deposits, 24, 26, 38
derivatives, 8, 10, 16, 102
dermal, 74, 76, 77, 78
dermatitis, 74, 85, 86, 87
dermatology, 70
dermis, 75
desorption, 11
destruction, 1, 3, 5, 6, 7, 70
dexamethasone, 86
diabetes, 42
differentiation, 4, 6, 13, 19, 22, 30, 44, 51, 52, 59, 60, 70, 78, 101, 107, 108, 113, 114
diffraction, 12
diffusion, 14, 75
dimeric, 54
dimerization, 50, 54
dinucleotides, 18, 73, 74
diphtheria, 12, 19, 36, 47, 100

discipline, 103
disease model, 107
disease progression, 28, 34
disease-free survival, 26
diseases, 31, 51, 56, 62, 74, 75, 83, 90, 91, 100, 103
disorder, 80, 81
distribution, 26, 39, 49, 50, 51
dominance, 60
donors, 93
dosage, 26, 44
dosing, 21
down-regulation, 13
drosophila, 50, 62
drug action, 49
drug delivery, 91
drugs, 23, 68, 78
dry, 80, 87
dsRNA, 50, 56
duration, 21
dust, 75, 81
dysregulation, 37, 59

E

E. coli, 8, 15, 19
E6, 9
E7, 9
ears, 80
economic, 46
eczema, 80, 81, 87
efficacy, 12, 13, 16, 17, 22, 23, 26, 28, 29, 35, 56, 57, 58, 66, 69, 99, 102, 105
election, 47
electroporation, 84
embryonic, 4
empowered, 59
emulsions, 14, 103
encapsulated, 26, 91
encephalomyelitis, 114
encoding, 30, 46
endocytosis, 6, 13, 15
endogenous, 4, 6, 86
endoplasmic reticulum, 20, 71
engagement, 7, 51, 56, 65
England, 67, 68, 72
English, 86
enteric, 19
enterprise, 100
envelope, 59, 91

environment, 75, 95, 103
environmental, 81
enzyme, 21, 55
enzymes, 55
eosinophilia, 2, 70, 87
eosinophils, 6, 80, 81
epidemiological, 89
epidermal, 77, 84, 86, 98
epidermal cells, 84
epidermal growth factor, 98
epidermis, 75, 78
epithelial cell, 35, 51, 55, 59, 65
epithelial ovarian cancer, 47
epitope, 15, 30, 33, 35, 95
epitopes, 5, 7, 8, 32, 35, 41, 90, 92
Epstein-Barr virus, 12
equilibrium, 93
erythrocyte, 93, 97
erythrocytes, 93
Escherichia coli, 45, 68
esophageal, 44
ester, 57, 58
ethanolamine, 93
etiologic factor, 87
Europe, 9, 103, 104
European, 65, 68, 69, 70, 71, 95, 99, 100, 102, 103, 104, 105
European Commission, 99, 100, 104, 105
European Union, 104
evidence, 3, 14, 20, 27, 34, 89, 90, 93
evolution, 101
exercise, 102
exogenous, 4, 6, 109
experimental autoimmune encephalomyelitis, 114
exposure, 3, 7, 11, 91, 94
extracellular, 50, 51, 52, 58, 86

F

failure, 23, 100
falciparum malaria, 68, 95, 97
family, 4, 49, 50, 51, 53, 54, 59, 60, 63
Fas, 6
FasL, 6
fatigue, 21, 34
fatty acid, 15, 17, 57, 58
fatty acids, 17
fax, 89
feedback, 22, 86

fever, 30, 34
fibroblast, 51
fibronectin, 16
flow, 100, 105
fluid, 11, 43, 44
fluorescence, 81
focusing, 103, 104
follicular, 22
follicular lymphoma, 22
Fox, 42
Foxp3, 26
France, 40
freedom, 103
FTIR spectroscopy, 12
funding, 100, 103, 104, 105
fungi, 21
fusion, 15, 69, 91
fusion proteins, 69

G

gastric, 19, 46
gastrin, 4, 19, 46
gastrointestinal, 38, 42, 59
gastrointestinal tract, 59
gel, 11
gene, 2, 4, 8, 23, 24, 26, 27, 28, 29, 37, 38, 39, 40, 42, 45, 46, 50, 52, 65, 91
gene expression, 65
gene transfer, 27, 37, 38, 42, 45, 91
generation, 11, 14, 21, 22, 36, 38, 54, 74, 79, 83, 84, 86, 91, 92, 101, 114
genes, 3, 26, 30, 49, 54, 63
genetic, 28
genetics, 70
genital warts, 17, 20, 59
germ line, 50
GlaxoSmithKline, 61, 105
glycans, 46
glycine, 46
glycolipids, 91
glycoprotein, 31, 46, 114
glycoproteins, 91
glycoside, 13, 40
glycosylated, 14, 38, 45
glycosylation, 4, 14, 31
glycosylphosphatidylinositol, 58
goals, 74
gonadotropin, 4
government, 104

Gram-negative, 57
Gram-positive, 57, 67
granulocyte, 8, 22, 26, 27, 37, 41, 44, 45, 46, 82
granzymes, 6
groups, 3, 12, 14, 29, 55, 61, 93, 103, 104, 109, 110, 111
growth, 3, 19, 21, 26, 29, 41, 46, 55, 74, 79, 92, 93, 94, 98
growth factor, 19, 41, 98
growth rate, 94

H

H. pylori, 10
H1, 114
H1N1, 9, 15, 91
H3N2, 59
HA1, 91
hairy cell leukemia, 41
harvest, 28
health, 89, 90, 100
heart, 45
heart transplantation, 45
heat, 2, 8, 15, 19, 20, 41, 45, 102, 110
heat shock protein, 2, 45
hemagglutinin, 15, 100
hematologic, 34
hematopoiesis, 108
hematopoietic, 22, 41, 49, 59
hematopoietic cells, 49
hematopoietic system, 59
heme, 65
heme oxygenase, 65
hepatitis, 17, 18, 39, 59, 61, 68, 70, 72, 84, 91, 96, 101
hepatitis B, 17, 18, 39, 61, 68, 72, 84, 101
hepatitis C, 59, 61, 70
hepatocellular, 4, 26, 40
hepatocellular cancer, 4
hepatocellular carcinoma, 26, 40
hepatocyte, 92, 94
hepatocytes, 93, 94
hepatoma, 68
HER2, 86
herpes, 12, 101, 106
herpes simplex, 12, 101, 106
heterodimer, 50, 54, 57
heterogeneous, 4, 32
high-risk, 30, 32, 38, 45
histological, 31, 80

HIV/AIDS vii, ix, 3, 14, 17, 19, 89, 95, 100, 101, 103
HIV-1, 3, 14, 95
homology, 50
hormone, 19, 22, 29, 37
host, 12, 28, 49, 51, 62, 68, 69, 91, 92, 94, 96, 98, 101, 108
house dust, 75, 81
human, 2, 4, 8, 9, 10, 11, 12, 13, 17, 18, 19, 26, 30, 31, 37, 38, 39, 40, 41, 42, 43, 45, 46, 51, 55, 59, 60, 62, 64, 65, 69, 70, 71, 77, 80, 87, 91, 92, 94, 97, 99, 100, 101, 102, 104
human chorionic gonadotropin, 4
human leukocyte antigen, 30
human neutrophils, 64
human papilloma virus, 17
humans, 8, 15, 18, 22, 50, 57, 59, 67, 89, 93, 95, 100, 102
humoral immunity, 6, 69, 90, 94
hydrogen, 93
hydroxide, 11, 12, 13, 35, 36, 44, 45, 49, 99, 100, 107, 108
hydroxyapatite, 12
hydroxyl, 12
hydroxyl groups, 12
hyperkeratosis, 80, 81
hypersensitivity, 16, 23, 27, 30, 107, 110, 114
hypersensitivity reactions, 27
hypertrophy, 82
hypothesis, 3, 28, 109

I

ice, 81, 82, 111
id, 43
identification, 58, 59, 90, 104
IFN-β, 52
IFNγ, 13, 17, 18, 35
IgE, 11, 12, 60, 73, 74, 75, 77, 80, 81, 87, 107, 109, 110, 114
IgG, 12, 17, 18, 23, 31, 32, 33, 34, 35, 40, 61, 93, 94, 109, 110
IL-1, 2, 5, 10, 11, 18, 21, 26, 35, 36, 43, 50, 51, 52, 53, 55, 56, 60, 73, 74, 77, 78, 81, 82, 83, 86, 107, 112, 113, 114
IL-10, 5, 77, 78, 82, 83, 86
IL-13, 6, 36, 74, 81
IL-15, 5
IL-17, 107, 112, 113, 114

IL-2, x, 2, 5, 6, 13, 20, 21, 25, 26, 27, 29, 35, 36, 40, 42, 47, 74, 86, 91, 107, 111
IL-4, 5, 11, 13, 19, 36, 74, 77, 81, 86, 110
IL-6, x, 5, 11, 57, 60, 74, 107, 108, 109, 110, 111, 112, 113, 114
IL-8, 13, 55
immune activation, 16, 28
immune cells, 13, 50, 63
immune memory, 92
immune reaction, 5, 107
immune response, 1, 2, 3, 4, 5, 6, 7, 8, 11, 12, 13, 14, 16, 17, 18, 19, 20, 22, 23, 26, 29, 31, 32, 33, 35, 37, 40, 41, 43, 44, 46, 47, 49, 51, 57, 58, 59, 61, 63, 64, 66, 69, 70, 73, 74, 75, 77, 78, 79, 80, 81, 82, 83, 85, 89, 90, 91, 92, 94, 95, 96, 99, 100, 104, 107, 108, 110, 113, 114
immune system, 1, 2, 3, 5, 6, 7, 11, 18, 19, 20, 23, 49, 50, 51, 54, 57, 58, 61, 67, 90, 91, 108
immune-suppressive, 83
immunity, 3, 5, 8, 12, 13, 20, 22, 27, 31, 36, 37, 38, 42, 44, 45, 49, 50, 54, 56, 62, 64, 66, 68, 69, 70, 71, 73, 74, 79, 83, 84, 87, 89, 90, 91, 92, 94, 95, 96, 99, 100, 101
immunization, 6, 7, 13, 15, 19, 26, 31, 32, 33, 34, 35, 38, 41, 43, 44, 51, 56, 74, 83, 84, 85, 93, 94, 95, 101, 104, 107, 108, 109, 110, 111, 112, 113
immunocompetence, 85
immunocompetent cells, 74, 77
immunocompromised, 19
immunodeficiency, 20
immunogen, 19, 38, 90, 92
immunogenicity, 1, 7, 9, 10, 13, 15, 23, 26, 30, 31, 33, 35, 39, 61, 68, 69, 72, 89, 90, 91, 92, 93, 94
immunoglobulin, 4, 12, 59, 100, 114
immunoglobulin G, 12, 59
immunohistochemistry, 47
immunological, 1, 4, 7, 9, 13, 18, 20, 23, 30, 31, 42, 45, 80
immunology, 62, 63, 65, 66, 67, 68, 69, 70, 71, 72, 99, 101
immunomodulation, 84
immunomodulator, 46
immunomodulatory, 14, 101
immunopathogenesis, 85
immunopathology, 105
immunoprecipitation, 57
immunostimulant, 14, 85

immunostimulatory, 10, 14, 15, 19, 26, 27, 28, 46, 61, 72, 73, 74, 99, 100, 101
immunosuppression, 45
immunosuppressive, 3, 77
immunotherapy, 16, 32, 36, 37, 38, 39, 41, 42, 43, 44, 45, 46, 49, 71, 74, 75, 82, 83
Immunotherapy, 39, 42, 45, 46, 72
implementation, 104
in vitro, 19, 20, 22, 43, 55, 59, 69, 85, 93, 94, 111, 112, 113
in vivo, 11, 19, 20, 31, 37, 38, 42, 43, 45, 55, 56, 65, 66, 73, 78, 83, 96, 113, 114
inactive, 54
incidence, 3
inclusion, 31, 92
indices, 94
inducer, 60, 77, 109
induction, 1, 4, 5, 6, 7, 12, 15, 16, 17, 21, 23, 26, 27, 28, 31, 35, 37, 42, 52, 53, 63, 68, 69, 71, 74, 77, 82, 83, 84, 86, 87, 91, 94, 96, 101, 108, 112, 114
industrial, 30
infection, 3, 6, 12, 21, 42, 54, 62, 64, 70, 86, 91, 94, 96, 101, 105
infections, 12, 22, 24, 60, 61, 65, 99, 100
infectious, 2, 3, 18, 31, 51, 56, 62, 66, 68, 69, 90, 91, 100, 101, 103
infectious disease, 2, 18, 31, 51, 56, 62, 66, 68, 69, 90, 100, 103
inflammation, 3, 6, 12, 14, 54, 69, 74, 81, 82, 101
inflammatory, 7, 15, 16, 20, 24, 35, 46, 53, 63, 69, 70, 74, 77, 80, 81, 101, 110, 114
inflammatory mediators, 110
inflammatory response, 7, 16, 24, 69, 70
inflammatory responses, 7, 70
influenza, 9, 13, 15, 16, 47, 59, 69, 71, 84, 89, 90, 91, 92, 94, 95, 96, 100, 101, 105
influenza a, 91
influenza vaccine, 9, 13, 69
inhibition, 2, 64, 85, 94
inhibitor, 54, 55, 70, 73, 77, 78, 79, 80, 83
inhibitors, 79
inhibitory, 3, 79, 86, 92, 93, 94, 97, 98
inhibitory effect, 79
initiation, 4, 6, 90
injection, 7, 11, 12, 13, 15, 17, 18, 23, 26, 27, 32, 34, 61, 100, 109, 111, 112
injections, 18, 23, 30, 32, 93
injuries, 81
injury, 65, 66

innate immunity, 54, 62, 64, 91
inoculation, 95
inoculum, 26
iNOS, 55
interaction, 5, 16, 19, 21, 54, 55, 57, 105
Interaction, 11
interactions, 5, 6, 57
interferon, 20, 21, 36, 37, 38, 40, 41, 44, 50, 52, 53, 63, 65, 66, 71, 101
interferon (IFN), 53
interferon gamma, 21, 44
interferons, 16
interleukin, 36, 37, 39, 41, 42, 43, 44, 45, 46, 51, 55, 62, 64, 66, 101, 108, 114
interleukin-1, 45, 51, 62, 66, 101
Interleukin-1, 66, 86
interleukin-2, 36, 37, 39, 41, 46
interleukin-6, 108, 114
interleukin-8, 55
interstitial, 11, 44
interval, 28
intervention, 80
intramuscular, 61
intramuscular injection, 61
intravascular, 43
intravenous, 21
intrinsic, 35, 90, 91
invasive, 37, 74, 76, 77, 79
investigative, 70
ionic, 8
ions, 11
ischaemia, 66
ischemia, 55, 65
isoelectric point, 11, 12
isolation, 42

J

Japan, 58, 73, 80, 107
Japanese, 80
Jefferson, 45
Jun, 66, 67, 68, 69, 70, 71, 72
Jung, 44, 45

K

kappa B, 65, 66, 69
killer cells, 21, 22
killing, 31

kinase, 53, 54, 55, 63, 64, 65, 84, 86
kinases, 53, 86
kinetics, 33
knockout, 77, 78, 86

L

labeling, 20
labor, 29
Langerhans cells, 21, 74, 76, 110
laser, 81
late-stage, 17
lead, 8, 11, 13, 27, 37, 53, 55, 57, 73, 74, 84, 101, 114
leakage, 21
lecithin, 15
lesions, 27, 70, 80, 81, 82, 83, 85, 87
leukemia, 20, 21, 22, 41, 59
leukemia cells, 59
leukocyte, 30, 64
leukocytosis, 28
liberation, 53, 54
life span, 64
life-threatening, 99, 100
ligand, 12, 21, 52, 56, 57, 59, 69, 70, 71, 101
ligands, 18, 49, 51, 53, 56, 60, 62, 69
likelihood, 28, 101
limitations, 100
linear, 90, 93
lipid, 8, 10, 15, 16, 17, 36, 50, 58, 68, 69, 91, 96, 101, 105
lipopolysaccharide, 8, 17, 57, 63, 64, 65, 67, 68, 71
lipoprotein, 50, 57, 64, 67
liposomes, 8, 10, 15, 25, 26, 40, 91, 92, 96
liquid chromatography, 68
listeria monocytogenes, 58, 70
literature, 90
liver, 20, 41, 44, 55, 92, 94, 96
liver metastases, 20
liver transplant, 44
liver transplantation, 44
L-lactide, 8
localization, 8, 54, 77, 81, 92
location, 26, 42, 50
locus, 4
long-term, 1, 31, 43, 45
LPS, 2, 8, 17, 49, 50, 53, 55, 57, 58, 64, 101
lung, 14, 28, 42, 44, 64, 65, 71, 86
lung cancer, 14, 28, 42, 71, 86

lungs, 55
lupus, 70
lymph, 5, 6, 13, 14, 41, 60, 71, 80, 81
lymph node, 5, 6, 13, 14, 41, 60, 71, 80, 81
lymphocyte, 27, 61, 66, 80
lymphocytes, 3, 13, 19, 21, 30, 37, 38, 42, 43, 46, 74, 80, 81, 84
lymphoid, 15, 74, 77
lymphoid organs, 15
lymphoid tissue, 74, 77
lymphoma, 21, 22
lymphomas, 3
lysine, 53
lysis, 5, 6, 31, 35, 79
lysosome, 71

M

mAb, 35, 37, 78
macrophage, 8, 22, 26, 27, 36, 37, 41, 44, 45, 46, 50, 51, 55, 57, 68, 80
macrophages, 5, 6, 11, 13, 20, 21, 27, 51, 55, 65, 67, 68, 73, 74, 77, 80, 81, 86, 91, 110
magnetic, 93
magnetic resonance, 93
maintenance, 16, 21
major histocompatibility complex, 38
malaise, 21
malaria, 14, 17, 68, 89, 92, 93, 94, 95, 96, 97, 98, 100, 103, 104
malignancy, 38, 42
malignant, 21, 36, 38, 42
malignant melanoma, 21
malignant tumors, 42
mammals, 8, 54
management, 9
manufacturing, 8, 103
marrow, 39, 59, 65, 70
mast cell, 80, 81
maturation, 6, 13, 22, 51, 57, 60, 66
maturation process, 6
Mcl-1, 64
MCP-1, 13
median, 21, 35, 39
mediators, 53, 67, 69, 78, 110
medicine, 56, 64, 65, 66, 67, 68, 70, 71, 72, 113
melanoma, 9, 10, 14, 17, 18, 20, 21, 23, 25, 26, 27, 28, 30, 36, 37, 38, 39, 40, 41, 43, 44, 45, 46, 47, 59, 70
membranes, 14, 91

memory, 26, 60, 71, 92, 94, 110
Merck, 17
meridian, 1
merozoites, 93, 98
metal salts, 11
metaphor, 96
metastases, 5, 20, 27, 58
metastasis, 6
metastatic, 17, 18, 20, 21, 27, 30, 32, 35, 39, 41, 43, 44, 45, 46, 70
metastatic cancer, 18, 39, 41
methicillin-resistant, 64
MHC class II molecules, 6, 11, 91
mice, 13, 19, 25, 26, 29, 37, 40, 42, 44, 47, 53, 55, 57, 58, 59, 63, 64, 67, 70, 73, 75, 76, 77, 78, 79, 80, 81, 82, 84, 85, 86, 87, 92, 93, 96, 107, 108, 109, 110, 111, 112, 113, 114
microbial, 10, 15, 17, 19, 24, 57, 58, 63, 66, 87
microenvironment, 23, 26, 90
microorganisms, 57, 62
microparticles, 26
microscope, 82
microscopy, 81
microspheres, 8, 24, 26
migration, 6, 13, 55, 60, 64, 78, 82, 83, 86, 94
military, 12, 102
mimicking, 7, 11, 90
mineral oils, 14, 49
mirror, 92
mites, 81
mitogen, 86
mitogen-activated protein kinase, 86
model system, 102
models, 4, 12, 13, 14, 18, 19, 22, 23, 26, 27, 31, 44, 58, 69, 89, 102, 107, 108, 112
modulation, 39
moieties, 90
molar ratio, 12
molecular biology, 61, 70, 102
molecular mechanisms, 41
molecular medicine, 64
molecular weight, 77, 81
molecules, 1, 2, 3, 4, 5, 6, 7, 11, 38, 49, 50, 53, 54, 56, 57, 90, 91, 92, 101
momentum, 100, 105
monkeys, 12, 33, 34, 35, 40, 93
monoclonal, 11, 35, 37, 43, 47, 61, 93
monoclonal antibodies, 11, 35, 37, 43, 47, 61, 93
monocyte, 13, 44, 55, 71
monocytes, 11, 13, 22, 45, 51, 59, 64, 80
monomeric, 58
mononuclear cell, 16, 91
monotherapy, 19, 61
morphology, 94
mouse, 19, 26, 27, 55, 64, 66, 68, 69, 75, 81, 84, 86, 87, 108, 112, 113, 114
mouse model, 19, 68, 86
mRNA, 11, 78, 80, 81, 82
mucin, 4, 14, 31, 32, 39, 41, 43
multicellular organisms, 50
multiple myeloma, 21
murine model, 12, 13, 27, 85
murine models, 12, 13, 27
muscle, 30
mutant, 59
mutants, 102
mutations, 3
myalgia, 17, 34
mycobacteria, 16, 57, 67, 107, 108, 110
myelin, 114
myelin oligodendrocyte glycoprotein, 114
myeloid, 22, 50, 51, 52, 59, 70, 101
myeloma, 21

N

N-acety, 44, 91
nanoparticles, 71
nanoparticulate, 12
national, 104
National Academy of Sciences, 67
natural, 4, 5, 6, 10, 12, 13, 14, 18, 20, 21, 31, 32, 45, 51, 68, 94, 95, 101, 110
natural killer, 5, 6, 21, 51
natural killer cell, 21, 22, 51
nausea, 21
neck, 80
necrosis, 27, 63, 68
neoplasias, 4, 37
neoplasms, 16
nervous system, 21
network, 6, 37, 77, 103
neuraminidase, 91
neutralization, 64
neutropenia, 22
neutrophil, 55, 64
neutrophilia, 55
neutrophils, 20, 22, 55, 64
New England, 67, 68, 72
New York, 13, 36, 63, 66, 67, 69

next generation, 36
NF-kB, 86
NF-κB, 52, 53, 54, 57
Nile, 59, 69
nitric oxide, 55, 65, 69, 86
nitric oxide synthase, 55, 69, 86
NK cells, 5, 16, 20, 35, 51, 74
nodes, 5, 6, 13, 14, 41, 60, 71
non toxic, 102
non-invasive, 74, 76, 77, 79
non-profit, 103
nontoxic, 58, 68, 69
normal, 4, 31, 53, 77, 111
not-for-profit, 104
N-terminal, 51, 93
nuclear, 53, 54, 57, 65
nuclear factor-κB, 53
nuclear magnetic resonance (NMR), 93
nucleic acid, 18, 71
nucleus, 54

O

observations, 35
oil, 2, 8, 9, 13, 14, 17, 103, 108
oils, 14, 49
oligodeoxynucleotides, viii, 8, 18, 39, 73, 74, 84, 85, 86, 87
oligomerization, 50, 52
oligonucleotides, 10, 18, 71, 87
oncogene, 4, 37, 64
oncology, 38
optical, 82
optimization, 92, 95, 97
oral, 10, 15, 101
oral polio vaccine, 102
organ, 3, 41, 54, 75
organism, 2
organizations, 100, 102, 103, 105
ovarian, 4, 21, 31, 32, 33, 39, 43, 47
ovarian cancer, 32, 39, 47
overproduction, 101
oxidative, 55, 64
oxide, 55, 65, 69, 86
oxygen, 54

P

P. falciparum, 92, 95

p53, 4, 42
pain, 17, 30
pancreatic, 19, 68
pancreatic cancer, 19
paper, 59
paracrine, 23, 24, 39, 66, 67
parameter, 15, 92
parasite, 89, 92, 93, 94, 95, 96, 97, 98
parasitemia, 94
parasites, 22, 55, 93, 94
parenteral, 15, 101
Parkinson, 43
particles, 8, 9, 11, 15, 92
passive, 35
pathogenesis, 74, 80, 85, 87
pathogenic, 114
pathogens, 18, 21, 49, 50, 51, 54, 56, 57, 58, 61, 62, 67, 90, 97, 99, 100, 101
pathology, 55, 74, 112
pathways, 6, 51, 52, 53, 55, 56, 62, 63, 64, 80, 91, 114
patients, 2, 3, 4, 11, 14, 16, 17, 18, 19, 20, 21, 22, 23, 27, 28, 29, 30, 31, 32, 33, 34, 35, 36, 37, 38, 39, 40, 41, 42, 43, 44, 45, 46, 59, 60, 61, 69, 70, 74, 75, 80, 81, 82, 83
pattern recognition, 49, 50, 58, 62, 67, 91
peptide, 4, 6, 8, 19, 20, 23, 29, 30, 31, 36, 42, 43, 44, 50, 59, 66, 83, 84, 90, 91, 92, 93, 94, 95, 96, 97, 98
peptides, 4, 6, 8, 20, 23, 30, 31, 37, 38, 61, 84, 89, 90, 91, 92, 93, 94, 95, 97
perforin, 5, 6
performance, 68, 102
peripheral blood, 11, 30, 64, 91
peripheral blood mononuclear cell, 91
peritoneal, 17, 33, 43
pH, 11, 12
phagocytic, 21
phagocytosis, 5, 6, 11, 55
pharmacokinetic, 21
pharmacokinetic parameters, 21
pharmacokinetics, 28
pharmacological, 58
pharmacology, 65, 69
phenotype, 4, 31, 58, 66, 71
phenotypic, 13
phone, 89
phosphate, 9, 11, 12, 36, 38, 40, 58, 85
phosphatidylcholine, 91
phosphatidylethanolamine, 91

phospholipids, 15, 91
phosphorylates, 54
phosphorylation, 54
physiological, 12, 26
physiology, 65, 70
pI, 11
PI3K, 55, 65, 66
pigs, 17
placebo, 19, 23, 41, 44
plasma, 27, 52, 59, 60, 70
plasma cells, 60
plasma membrane, 52
plasmid, 10, 84
plasmodium falciparum, 68, 89, 95, 97, 98
play, 4, 6
pneumonia, 55, 65
Poland, 39
policy makers, 100, 105
polio, 102
polymer, 8, 26
polymers, 8
polypeptide, 91
polysaccharide, 14
poor, 4, 31, 61, 89, 100, 102
poor performance, 102
population, 90, 112
power, 9
pragmatic, 103
preclinical, 2, 17, 26, 27, 28, 93, 95, 104
pre-existing, 12, 26, 92, 94, 95
preparation, 14, 104
prevention, 91
primary tumor, 16, 26
primate, 44, 69
primates, 9
priming, 5, 6, 7, 26, 28, 36, 39, 42, 56, 61, 66, 77, 83, 84, 86
private, 102, 103
private enterprises, 102
private sector, 102
probe, 14
procedures, 74, 90
production, 12, 13, 14, 18, 21, 30, 36, 38, 50, 55, 56, 57, 59, 60, 65, 68, 70, 73, 74, 75, 77, 78, 81, 82, 84, 86, 107, 108, 109, 110, 111, 112, 113, 114
profit, 103, 104
progenitor cells, 59, 70
progenitors, 22
prognosis, 4, 16, 31, 39
progressive, 30
proinflammatory, 15, 16, 20, 21, 35, 54, 55, 59, 63, 65, 67, 69, 74, 77
proinflammatory effect, 55
proliferation, 19, 55, 60, 70, 83, 94, 108
promote, 6, 7, 8, 19, 22, 26, 53, 83, 90
property, 99, 100
prophylactic, 2, 3, 27, 40, 51, 56, 96, 106
prophylaxis, 74, 79
prostaglandin, 77, 86, 87
prostate, 4, 14, 22, 29, 31, 37, 43, 45
prostate cancer, 14, 22, 29, 37, 45
prostate carcinoma, 29
prostate specific antigen, 4
prostatitis, 16
proteases, 54
protection, 3, 9, 12, 17, 26, 28, 40, 45, 51, 56, 59, 66, 90, 92, 93, 94, 96, 101, 105
protein, 2, 4, 6, 11, 12, 16, 17, 18, 19, 20, 31, 33, 35, 40, 41, 43, 45, 46, 50, 52, 53, 54, 58, 59, 62, 66, 68, 69, 84, 86, 89, 90, 92, 93, 95, 96, 97, 98, 101
protein kinases, 53, 86
proteins, 3, 4, 7, 8, 11, 14, 15, 20, 30, 42, 45, 49, 50, 51, 52, 54, 57, 58, 61, 68, 69, 89, 90, 91, 92, 94, 97, 99, 101
proteoglycans, 96
proteolysis, 54
protocol, 94
protocols, 27, 45, 60, 102
Pseudomonas, 55, 65
Pseudomonas aeruginosa, 65
public, 89, 90, 100, 102, 103
public domain, 103
public health, 89, 90, 100
public sector, 102, 103
pulse, 30
purification, 58
pyrimidine, 54

R

radiation, 59
radiotherapy, 59
range, 15, 90, 102
ras, 4
rat, 68
rats, 59, 71
reactive oxygen species, 54
reactivity, 15, 31, 32, 35, 43

reagents, 62
receptor agonist, 69
receptors, 7, 17, 18, 49, 50, 53, 56, 58, 59, 62, 63, 64, 67, 70, 71, 91, 99, 101
recognition, 2, 3, 7, 31, 41, 49, 50, 57, 58, 62, 64, 67, 91, 97, 98, 101
recruiting, 22
recurrence, 21, 40, 47
redistribution, 94
reduction, 11, 70
refractory, 22, 29, 37, 70
regional, 23, 74, 77
regression, 23, 24, 26, 30, 37, 41, 58, 68, 85, 86
regular, 4
regulation, 13, 15, 22, 64, 65, 66, 71, 74, 78, 81, 83
regulations, 82
regulators, 4
regulatory requirements, 30
rejection, 28, 45, 68
relapse, 30, 32, 69
relationship, 11
remission, 33
remodeling, 71
renal, 21, 42, 43, 46
renal cell carcinoma, 21, 42, 43
reperfusion, 55, 65, 66
repression, 65
research, 63, 66, 68, 71, 97, 99, 100, 102, 103, 104, 105
research and development, 97, 100, 103, 105
research funding, 100, 105
researchers, 102
resection, 16, 26, 41
residues, 15, 54, 57, 93
resistance, 22, 55, 65, 66, 68
resources, 103
respiratory, 55, 71
responsiveness, 2, 86
reticulum, 20, 71
retroviral, 38
rheumatoid arthritis, 55, 111
rhinitis, 72
Rho, 81
risk, 4, 22, 30, 32, 33, 38, 45, 101, 102
rituximab, 22
rodents, 93
Rössler, 40

S

safety, 2, 17, 18, 29, 30, 33, 36, 39, 72, 90, 91, 93, 94, 101, 102, 103, 105
saline, 61, 108, 109
salmonella, 17, 58, 59, 68, 69
salt, 9, 14
salts, 2, 8, 9, 11, 103
sample, 9
saponin, 8, 9, 14, 15, 31, 45
saponins, 9, 15
sarcomas, 3
saturation, 27
scatter, 33
scientific, 29, 89, 100, 103, 105
scientists, 56, 62
search, 103, 105
Seattle, 103
secrete, 22, 27, 28, 37, 44, 45, 54, 74, 84
secretin, 28, 37
secretion, 2, 13, 19, 20, 27, 28, 60, 66, 73, 74, 84, 114
self, 34
sensitivity, 92
sensors, 62
sequelae, 7
serine, 44, 54, 98
serum, 11, 33, 34, 35, 43, 61, 80, 94, 110, 111, 112
severity, 10
sharing, 28
shock, 2, 8, 20, 41, 42, 43, 45
sialic acid, 15
side effects, 8, 21, 23, 32, 61
signaling, 6, 36, 44, 51, 52, 53, 54, 57, 58, 59, 62, 63, 64, 65, 67, 68, 87, 101, 105, 107
signaling pathway, 51, 52, 53, 62, 63, 64, 67
signaling pathways, 51, 52, 53, 62, 63, 64
signalling, 62, 63
signals, 4, 6, 7, 8, 42, 49, 53, 54, 57, 62, 66, 71, 81, 86, 101
signs, 20
similarity, 51, 92
Singapore, 9, 91
sites, 5, 6, 14, 25, 27, 32, 54, 62, 76, 83
skeleton, 10, 17
skin, 6, 21, 27, 32, 73, 74, 75, 76, 77, 78, 79, 80, 81, 82, 83, 84, 85, 87, 110
skin-associated lymphoid tissue, 74, 77
smallpox, 100

sodium, 58
solid tumors, 23
solubility, 77
sorting, 35
spatial, 39
species, 10, 54, 92, 97
specificity, 63, 96
spectroscopy, 12, 93
spleen, 79, 107, 111, 112, 113
sporadic, 14
stability, 14
stages, 16, 41, 89, 94, 95, 96
stakeholders, 100, 103, 105
Staphylococcus aureus, 55, 64
stem cell transplantation, 36
sterile, 2, 94
stimulant, 22
stomach, 19
strain, 58, 80, 91, 102
strains, 87
strategies, 3, 16, 62, 77, 85
subcutaneous tissue, 75
sub-Saharan Africa, 92
subtilisin, 93
sugar, 58
sulfate, 96
sulphate, 58
superficial bladder cancer, 16
superiority, 32
supernatant, 112
superoxide, 55
suppression, 1, 3, 56, 57, 66, 68, 74, 78, 81
suppressor, 4
suppressors, 26
surface structure, 90
surfactant, 9, 14
surfactants, 8
surgery, 16, 20, 49
surgical, 16
surgical resection, 16
surveillance, 3, 37
survival, 3, 4, 16, 17, 19, 20, 21, 26, 28, 30, 31, 32, 35, 40, 41, 47, 55
susceptibility, 55
Sweden, 99
swelling, 110, 111
Switzerland, 89, 93
symptoms, 21, 32, 59, 61, 70, 74, 112
syndrome, 20, 21
synergistic, 23, 27, 56

synergistic effect, 23, 27, 56
synthesis, 14, 40, 53, 57, 60, 65, 90, 97
synthetic, 2, 10, 14, 17, 18, 19, 30, 31, 32, 35, 38, 39, 41, 43, 45, 57, 59, 60, 61, 68, 69, 73, 74, 84, 89, 90, 91, 92, 93, 94, 95, 96, 97
systems, 7, 8, 49, 89, 99, 100, 102

T

T cell, 1, 2, 3, 4, 5, 6, 7, 11, 15, 18, 19, 20, 22, 23, 24, 27, 28, 30, 37, 39, 41, 42, 43, 44, 45, 47, 50, 51, 56, 57, 60, 61, 66, 71, 73, 74, 77, 78, 82, 84, 86, 87, 90, 91, 92, 93, 94, 95, 96, 99, 100, 107, 108, 110, 112, 113, 114
T lymphocyte, 13, 19, 37, 38, 46, 74, 80
T lymphocytes, 13, 19, 37, 38, 46, 74, 80
T regulatory cells, 36, 56
Tanzania, 94
targets, 3, 4, 31, 47, 49, 59, 80
technology, 33, 35
telomerase, 4
temperature, 92
testes, 4
testis, 30, 31
tetanus, 8, 12, 19, 23, 30, 36, 44, 47, 100
therapeutic, 2, 3, 16, 17, 21, 23, 27, 40, 51, 56, 59, 80, 96, 106
therapeutics, 1, 63
therapy, 1, 2, 3, 4, 14, 16, 21, 22, 23, 31, 32, 35, 37, 43, 61, 71, 74, 77, 79, 87
thermal, 12
thermal analysis, 12
threatening, 99, 100, 103
threonine, 44
thymocytes, 108
time, 7, 28, 32, 37, 81, 89, 93, 100, 102, 105, 113
tissue, 6, 7, 8, 11, 13, 26, 74, 75, 77
TLR2, 49, 50, 53, 55, 57, 63, 64, 67, 69
TLR3, 50, 51, 52, 53, 55, 60
TLR4, 49, 50, 51, 53, 55, 57, 58, 63, 64, 65, 68, 101, 105
TLR9, 18, 19, 39, 44, 49, 50, 51, 53, 60, 61, 70, 71, 72, 84, 101
T-lymphocytes, 30, 42, 84
TNF-α, 58
Tokyo, 73, 87
tolerance, 1, 5, 6, 9, 12, 31, 38, 42, 56, 66, 67, 68
toll-like, 18, 63, 64, 65, 67, 69, 70, 71, 72, 73, 74, 77, 105
toxic, 1, 2, 3, 10, 23, 58, 68, 102

Index

toxicities, 30, 32, 59
toxicity, 2, 9, 10, 14, 15, 16, 21, 22, 23, 29, 32, 57, 58, 59, 102
toxin, 3, 8, 15, 19, 38, 42, 45, 102, 105
toxins, 8, 10, 19, 42, 61, 63, 102
training, 103
trans, 80, 93
transcription, 54, 57
transcription factor, 54, 57
transduction, 24, 28
transfection, 29
transfer, 27, 36, 37, 38, 42, 45, 68, 91
transgenic, 19, 42
transgenic mice, 42
translational, 104
translocation, 54, 65
transmembrane, 51, 58, 93
transplant, 22, 32
transplantation, 3, 36, 44, 45
transport, 92
Tregs, 56, 82, 83
trend, 32, 61
trial, 12, 14, 16, 17, 19, 20, 21, 23, 26, 27, 28, 29, 30, 32, 33, 37, 39, 40, 42, 43, 44, 46, 59, 61, 70, 94, 95, 96, 98, 101, 105
triggers, 54, 85
tuberculosis, 17, 67, 89, 100, 104, 108
tumor, 1, 2, 3, 4, 5, 6, 7, 8, 12, 16, 18, 19, 20, 21, 22, 23, 24, 25, 26, 27, 28, 29, 30, 31, 32, 33, 34, 35, 37, 38, 39, 40, 41, 42, 43, 44, 45, 46, 47, 56, 58, 59, 63, 66, 68, 69, 73, 74, 75, 77, 79, 83, 84, 85
tumor associated antigens, 3, 26
tumor cells, 2, 3, 4, 5, 6, 7, 8, 16, 20, 24, 25, 26, 27, 28, 31, 32, 33, 34, 35, 37, 38, 40, 41, 42, 44, 79
tumor growth, 3, 74, 79
tumor metastasis, 6
tumor necrosis factor, 63, 68
tumor progression, 21, 28
tumorigenesis, 86
tumors, 2, 3, 17, 23, 25, 26, 28, 29, 31, 37, 40, 41, 42, 43, 44, 45, 46, 58, 77
typhoid, 102

U

Ubiquitin, 54, 63
ultrasound, 68
United States, 67
urease, 10
urine, 11, 37, 51

V

vaccination, 1, 3, 6, 11, 12, 13, 14, 16, 17, 19, 20, 22, 23, 25, 26, 27, 28, 29, 30, 31, 32, 34, 36, 40, 41, 42, 43, 46, 56, 57, 60, 61, 62, 66, 67, 73, 74, 75, 76, 77, 78, 79, 83, 84, 85, 90, 94, 95, 101
vaccinations, 17, 18, 25, 30, 32, 99
vaccine, 1, 2, 4, 6, 7, 9, 10, 11, 12, 13, 14, 15, 16, 17, 18, 19, 20, 22, 23, 26, 28, 29, 30, 31, 32, 33, 34, 35, 36, 37, 38, 39, 40, 41, 42, 43, 44, 45, 46, 47, 51, 56, 57, 58, 59, 60, 61, 62, 66, 68, 69, 70, 72, 74, 76, 77, 79, 83, 89, 90, 91, 92, 93, 94, 95, 96, 97, 98, 99, 100, 101, 102, 103, 104, 105
vaccines, 1, 2, 3, 4, 7, 8, 9, 11, 12, 13, 14, 22, 23, 24, 26, 27, 28, 29, 30, 31, 32, 34, 35, 36, 37, 38, 39, 41, 43, 44, 45, 46, 47, 49, 51, 56, 57, 60, 61, 66, 73, 74, 83, 89, 90, 91, 92, 94, 96, 99, 100, 101, 102, 103, 104, 105, 106, 108
Valencia, 38
vascular, 21
vasculature, 101
vector, 4, 6, 28, 38
vertebrates, 50
vessels, 6
viral, 4, 6, 8, 9, 15, 18, 42, 49, 50, 55, 59, 60, 61, 63, 91, 96
viral diseases, 91
viral vectors, 8
virus, 8, 12, 15, 17, 23, 30, 42, 46, 59, 61, 66, 69, 70, 84, 91, 92, 96, 101, 105, 106
virus infection, 42, 96, 105
viruses, 21, 70, 90
visual, 112
vitiligo, 25
voice, 103
vomiting, 21

W

warts, 17, 20, 59
waste, 103
water, 2, 9, 13, 14, 16, 17, 40, 77, 103, 108
water-soluble, 40
Watson, 3, 38, 46

web, 1
weight loss, 21
Weinberg, 86
West Nile virus, 59, 69
women, 32
workers, 58
World Health Organization, 40, 104

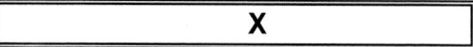

xenograft, 26
X-ray, 12

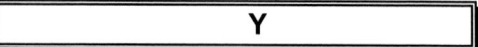

yield, 30